ROOTED

Rooted

The Hidden Cause of Disease and How to Heal Naturally

Dr. Sierra Bains

Published by Game Changer Publishing
Cover Design by Futurum

Paperback ISBN: 978-1-967424-13-9
Hardcover ISBN: 978-1-967424-14-6
Digital ISBN: 978-1-967424-15-3

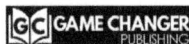

GC GAME CHANGER PUBLISHING
www.GameChangerPublishing.com

DEDICATION

To you, the reader,

For the days you felt dismissed, the symptoms that stole your spirit, and the system that made you question your own sanity.

For the version of me who lived there too, searching, spiraling, and still standing.

This book is a reclamation. A return. A handbook home to the wisdom that has always been yours, so you never have to outsource your knowing again.

With deep gratitude.

Dr. Sierra

READ THIS FIRST

As a thank you for investing in your health, I've created
a collection of free resources to support your journey.

Download Them Here:

ROOTED

THE HIDDEN CAUSE OF DISEASE AND HOW TO HEAL NATURALLY

DR. SIERRA BAINS

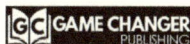

GC GAME CHANGER
PUBLISHING
www.GameChangerPublishing.com

CONTENTS

From Bodybuilder to Bedridden 1

Chapter 1 – The Flawed Foundation 9

Chapter 2 – Wired for Wellness 23

Chapter 3 – Mastering Your Metabolism...............................37

Chapter 4 – Food For Thought 49

Chapter 5 – Living in Sync...67

Chapter 6 – Let's Talk About Sex (Hormones)......................83

Chapter 7 – Movement Is Medicine.....................................105

Chapter 8 – The Invisible Disease 117

Chapter 9 – The Stress Factor 131

Chapter 10 – Back to Basics...141

The Rooted Return 143

Conclusion..151

References...153

FROM BODYBUILDER TO BEDRIDDEN

"It has been years since I have delivered one of these diagnoses," my doctor stated coldly. "You have multiple sclerosis."

My chest tightened, my body shook, and hot tears spilled down my 24-year-old face as her words sank in like a punch to the gut.

Multiple sclerosis (MS) is a relentless autoimmune disease that targets the brain and spinal cord, often stealing one's strength, focus, and ability to move freely. MS was also my doctor's unsettling explanation for the nerve pain, migraines, numbness, tingling, bleeding, confusion, and brain lesions that suddenly developed just one month prior.

In graduate school, I learned about MS from a doctor who had suffered with it. She was hardly over 50, yet had already been dependent on a wheelchair. Now, staring at my diagnosis, I pictured myself following the same path: losing my mobility over the next two decades.

As a lifelong competitive athlete, bodybuilder, and physical therapy student, movement was not just something I did. It was who I was. MS could not be the end of my story. I would not accept it.

For the next several months, I traveled across the United States in search of answers. I found myself constantly seated in a sterile waiting room, clutching clipboards full of intake forms, repeating my symptoms to doctor after doctor. After every visit, I clung to a thread of hope as a new specialist walked in, only to leave with another prescription, another shrug, and another referral to someone else. Meanwhile, my daily battle with symptoms raged on with intense migraines blurring my vision, stabbing nerve sensations with every step, and full-body tingling that stole my sleep. I fought to keep up with my doctorate program, but I was no longer a "normal" student. My life had become a revolving door of unanswered questions, temporary fixes, and the sinking realization that no one was truly connecting the dots.

While my classmates attended lectures, I endured invasive nerve conduction studies with tiny needles zapping my muscles. While others took exams in groups, I lay flat on a desk, battling the complications of a spinal tap that left me unable to sit up for weeks. The spinal fluid supporting my brain had leaked out, leaving me with debilitating nausea and pain. For my typically active body to now be dormant, it was nothing short of hell.

After dozens of tests, I was offered only one solution: a black box drug. Black Box Warnings are the most serious from the Food and Drug Administration (FDA), reserved for medications that carry life-threatening effects, including suicidal ideation. My doctor told me I would need to take the drug every day for the rest of my life to mitigate my misery.

I remember reluctantly picking up the pharmaceutical on my way home from class. At the time, I was also an intermittent cannabis user to manage my pain. That day, with nerves on fire and tears welling in my eyes, I entered my apartment and sank onto the stool at my kitchen counter.

In one hand, I held the prescription bottle. In the other, a joint I had left out earlier. My future flashed before me as I contemplated taking the first pill of thousands I would end up relying on to manage my neurological symptoms. That reality felt like defeat, and I was not ready to give in. I shook my head, threw the bottle in the trash, and reached for a lighter.

MY AWAKENING

Before my diagnosis, my future felt certain. I had planned my path: go to school, become a doctor, and dedicate my life to serving others. I obeyed rules without question, attended the highest-ranked programs, and consistently performed at the top of my class.

Multiple sclerosis was not a part of my perfect plan and forced me to confront the most important question of my life: *Why?* Why had I abruptly gotten so sick despite being in the best shape of my life? Why was medication my only option? Why were my doctors so unwilling to discuss causes and alternatives? How had I gone from consistently outperforming men in the gym to struggling just to drive my car?

When one doctor did not have an answer, I was sent to another. I became a regular at my primary care physician's, the neurologist's office, and the pain clinic. I do not fault those medical professionals. I believe they were doing their best with the tools they were given. Unfortunately, those tools view the body as separate parts rather than the whole, leading to endless appointments with few solutions.

As I cycled through providers, the truth hit me hard. The healthcare system was not built to heal me. It was built to profit from my illness. The average annual expense for an individual with MS is $88,487.[1] Given how young I was, that was an inevitable $4 million in prescriptions, doctor visits, hospitalizations, and other medical services throughout my life. There was more money to be made in keeping me sick than in helping me heal.

I knew something was not adding up. Not just in my case, but for the countless cases I would eventually support. I did not want to cover up my symptoms with a pill. I wanted to resolve them for good.

Slowly, I began to piece things together. In the months leading up to my diagnosis, I was training intensely for a bodybuilding competition. As a bodybuilder, I was striving for peak fitness and meticulously tracking all aspects of my day. I monitored my foods, workouts, and biomarkers. I was at a healthy weight and in the best physical shape of my life.

The only notable change from my candidly mundane routine came on February 8, 2021, when I received my second dose of the Pfizer COVID-19 vaccine. On February 9th, I experienced my first neurological symptoms.

At the time, the world was reeling from the pandemic, which had already claimed millions of lives. Vaccines were hastily rolled out in an effort to curb mortality rates. As a graduate student on a hospital rotation, it was mandatory to get vaccinated for COVID-19 to maintain my role and academic standing. I did not question it. Like many in healthcare, I was conditioned to follow medical protocols with blind trust.

One late night in search of information, I stumbled across the work of Dr. Robert Malone, an early pioneer of mRNA technology (used in the COVID-19 vaccines) and a vocal critic of the management of the pandemic. He raised concerns about the potential for these vaccines to cross the blood-brain barrier, leading to neurological damage.

As I read more, my suspicions grew. *Could the vaccine have been the major player in my rapid decline?* Each time I raised the possibility with my providers, I was dismissed. There were no questions, no curiosity. Just fast denials.

Conventional healthcare had no roadmap for me, so I needed to look elsewhere. In my hundreds of hours of research, I discovered a different approach: functional medicine. Unlike the standard system, which prescribes a pill in response to a diagnosis, this root-cause method seeks to understand lifestyle, nutrition, and stressors to help the whole body operate optimally.

In a matter of months, I used functional practices to learn *why* I had gotten sick, help my system process the lingering effects of the vaccine, and resolve every symptom on my own. The tingling started to skip days, then weeks, and then it subsided altogether. I regained my bubbly energy and sharp focus. I walked into the gym and could finally complete a leg workout without pain. And most importantly, I began to understand that vaccine injury was not the sole cause of my symptoms. For years, hidden stress had been building within me like a bomb waiting to detonate. Chronic inflammation, toxic exposure, and emotional burdens created imbalances that left me vulnerable to disease. A 1969 study done on thirty-two MS patients revealed that 85% of diagnoses were given in the wake of highly stressful events, whether family challenges or a sudden threat they deemed impossible to manage.[2] The vaccine administered to me in the middle of a global pandemic was neither the beginning nor the end of my story—it was the final straw in an already overwhelmed system.

THE ROOT CAUSE

If a tree is withering, you would not waste time trimming the branches or spraying the leaves. You would probably dig deeper and look at the roots because the health of the whole tree begins there, hidden underground, where no one can see. The same applies to you.

Many of us miss this truth because we were never shown another way. Instead, we spend years desperately trying to hold branches together with duct tape by chasing the latest fad diet, cycling through medications, and searching endlessly for answers that never seem to add up.

Merriam-Webster defines medicine as "the science and art dealing with the maintenance of health and prevention, alleviation, or the cure of disease." Somewhere along the way, we lost the art. We have reduced healthcare to a series of prescriptions that quiet symptoms, rather than a path that restores balance. The current system was built to manage illness, not resolve it, focusing on band-aid treatments instead of the deep, layered healing we truly need.

This book is here to change that.

You are not broken. You did not fail because you did not try hard enough. Your answers are not missing. They have simply been buried beneath the surface, waiting to be uncovered. Through my own journey and years of helping others, I have learned that at the core of every chronic condition lies one common root cause: nervous system dysregulation.

Your nervous system dictates everything, including when you take action, when you rest, and how your body responds to stress. Unfortunately, in today's world, most of us live in a state of chronic overload. Physical, emotional, and environmental stressors pile on, leaving our bodies stuck in a survival mode they were never designed to maintain.

These stressors come in many forms. External factors like over-exercising, a toxic environment, or ongoing family conflicts add up. Internal triggers such as gut issues, anxiety, or unresolved trauma amplify the damage. Even positive stress—like drive and ambition—is not immune to burnout. Without recovery, even your dreams can drain you.

Over time, chronic stress wreaks havoc. It floods your system with cortisol, drives inflammation, disrupts your hormones, and leaves your metabolism struggling to keep up. What starts as subtle signals, like poor sleep or feeling "off," can snowball until the symptoms feel unbearable.

This cycle does not own you. You have the power to break it and heal.

Real medicine begins with understanding what is throwing your body out of balance and taking intentional steps to restore alignment. You do not need a cabinet full of bottles or another exhausting list of things to cut out of your life. What you *do* need is the right foundation rooted in both science and the ancient wisdom of your body to help your nervous system find equilibrium again.

That is exactly what this book is here to teach you. Together, we will dive into the fundamentals you never learned in health class (but should have), like how the food system impacts your energy, the connection between fertility and your brain, how to recover deeply, why light and movement matter, and how stress subtly shapes your well-being.

You do not need a medical degree to understand it all, and I promise I am not going to ask you to give up chocolate, because that would be an unnecessary cruelty. I am here to heal, not harm. Whether you are looking to break free from years of struggle, prevent illness before it starts, or are ready to finally stop spiraling through the midnight symptom searches on Dr. Google, this is your guide.

Holistic practice is not just an alternative. It is the foundation for optimal health. It reconnects you with the strength and vitality you have always harbored. Imagine waking up each day feeling clear-headed, energized, and resilient, knowing your body is working for you, not against you.

We all want to feel healthy, not just for the sake of it, but because it fuels everything else we care about. Whether it is showing up fully in your relationships, building something meaningful, or advancing in your career, you need a body that can support the life you are here to create. Health is not a luxury. It is a requirement for sustainable success.

My intention with this book is to give you the simple tools to access that higher version of yourself, not just to feel better but to live with a sense of joy, clarity, and purpose that feels completely natural.

This is not wishful thinking. It is your intuition calling you home. And it starts here, at the roots.

CHAPTER 1

THE FLAWED FOUNDATION

"The greatest medicine of all is to teach
people how to not need it."
– Hippocrates

What if your "healthiest" habits are actually the ones making you sick? For Sophia, this was not a theoretical question. It was her harsh reality.

Sophia did not cut corners. She trained with intensity, logged every bite of food, and somehow managed to run a thriving business while also raising two little kids. She made it look easy, even enviable. From the outside, she was the definition of discipline, the woman others looked to for proof that balance was possible.

Underneath the polished routine, her health was starting to unravel. Even after nine hours of sleep, Sophia woke up groggy, like her body had missed the memo that rest was supposed to restore her. The kind of exhaustion she felt was bone-deep, the kind that coffee cannot touch and sleep cannot fix.

What Sophia did not know, and what most of us overlook, is that the health advice she followed was part of the problem. Her nervous system was fried, stuck in survival mode, and no amount of willpower was going to pull her out of it.

THE SILENT STRUGGLE

Sophia's crash did not come all at once. It crept in slowly, disguised as normal wear and tear of a full life. She was tired, sure, but who wasn't? *That is the price you pay when you are doing hard things,* she rationalized to herself to keep pushing.

By mid-morning, she had already downed her third cup of coffee just to stay upright. After her first pregnancy, the caffeine stopped working. Even with dialed-in meals and workouts that left her sweaty and breathless, the baby weight clung on like it had nowhere else to be. Every Sunday, she stepped onto the scale, holding her breath. And every Sunday, the number stared back unchanged.

The woman in the mirror started to feel like a stranger: softer, duller, like life had drained the color from her face. Then her hair started falling out. Not just a little extra shedding, but thick clumps, collecting in the shower drain. That is when she realized something was wrong, very wrong. She picked up the phone and called her doctor.

The diagnosis was hypothyroidism, a condition where the thyroid does not produce enough hormones. Her doctor blamed it for the fatigue, the weight gain, and her sluggish metabolism. He scribbled out prescriptions for levothyroxine and hormone replacement therapy, promising they would help. And at first, they did. Sophia's mental fog lifted, until it returned thicker and heavier. Migraines started crashing into her afternoons, bloating hit nearly every evening,

THE FLAWED FOUNDATION

and an additional fifteen pounds crept on, despite following a meal plan like religion.

Frustrated, Sophia returned to her doctor. His advice? Slash her calories to 1,400 a day and add a weight-loss medication to the mix. She followed the protocol with precision, but her body still did not respond.

Like so many left without answers, Sophia took matters into her own hands and turned to the internet. She became obsessed with scrolling forums, listening to podcasts, and ordering supplements she could not pronounce. She was not looking for a quick fix anymore. She just needed something that made sense. Her clothes no longer fit, her confidence cracked, and her sense of control vanished.

Life did not stop, but she struggled to participate. Sophia went through the motions of birthday parties, family dinners, and client calls, but it all felt forced. The sound of her kids laughing felt far away. Intimacy with her husband had faded. Her work, once her passion, now felt like a performance she couldn't keep up.

Defeated and disengaged, Sophia visited her doctor one more time. He added an antidepressant, not because he was sure she was depressed, but because he did not know what else to do. She took the prescription, but the emptiness remained. By the time Sophia came to me, she was at her breaking point, ready to try anything different.

STARTING FROM SCRATCH

From the moment we began, it was obvious no one had ever asked the most important question about Sophia's health: *Why?* Why was

11

she exhausted all the time? Why wasn't her body changing, no matter how hard she tried? Why had her symptoms stacked up despite multiple medications?

Sophia's experience was not unique. Like so many others, she had spent years bouncing between specialists, each one focused on a single symptom, but none of them seeing the full picture. Modern medicine was built to specialize, not to integrate. The deeper a provider focuses on one organ, the easier it becomes to lose sight of the human behind it. Sophia's fatigue was treated separately from weight gain. Bloating got its own diagnosis. Low libido was chalked up to hormones. Each issue was labeled, medicated, and boxed up, as if they came from different bodies. Nobody had paused to ask about her lifestyle, environment, and the subtle stressors that do not show up on a lab report but change everything about how the body functions.

I told Sophia what I tell nearly every client: treating fatigue with a medication is like putting tape over the check engine light and pretending the car is fine. You can ignore the warning, but eventually, it breaks down.

Our first consultation lasted over 90 minutes, during which we traced her full story, not just the recent flare-ups. We zoomed out to see that her symptoms had not been random. They were signals, connected, compounding, and pointing back to the same root imbalance. Our job was to uncover what threw her system out of alignment and start rebuilding from the ground up.

What we uncovered was telling. Sophia was consuming nearly 1,000 milligrams of caffeine a day, the equivalent of eight to ten cups of coffee! While caffeine offers a short-lived boost, Sophia's level overwhelmed her nervous system, leaving it depleted and dependent.

Her meals were convenient but hollow. Most days started with instant oats or a protein bar, easy to log, but hard to recover from. They lacked the nourishment her cells craved. She spent her days indoors, working behind screens, exercising under artificial lights, and disconnected from the sun. Without consistent exposure to natural light, the body's internal clock had lost its anchor.

Sophia was not simply tired. Her body had been stuck in survival mode for years, burning through reserves, trying to hold the line under nonstop stress.

FUNCTIONAL FOUNDATIONS

She was willing to do the work. What she needed first was clarity. We started with education. I explained how her screen-heavy lifestyle had slowly detached her from her brain's natural rhythm and it was critical for her energy and hormones. We moved away from her rigid tracking and built meals around nourishment and blood sugar balance.

Sophia's undeniable progress started before her lab results came in. Within a month, she had reduced her caffeine intake to zero, which was no small feat, given her starting point. Her energy returned, not in highs and crashes, but something she could rely on. Her hair stopped falling out in clumps, and for the first time in years, she began to feel like herself again.

When her lab results arrived, they validated what her symptoms had already told us both. Years of chronic stress had forced her body into self-preservation. She had developed what is known as a calcium shell: a mineral barrier that forms when the body pulls calcium from the bones to buffer against stress. The same shell meant to shield her cells also trapped toxins inside and blocked nutrients from getting in where they were needed. The system trying to save her had also slowed her ability to heal. Sitting with that realization, Sophia finally processed what her body had endured. Her symptoms were a cumulative effect of a system at war with itself.

A FRACTURED SYSTEM

Every day, I speak with people just like Sophia, who are diligent, proactive, and still trapped in the taxing loop of disease management. They have done everything short of a rain dance and still feel like hot garbage.

No amount of self-control can outpace a system designed to manage symptoms instead of solving them. While modern medicine excels in urgent situations like broken bones and treating life-threatening infections, it falls painfully short with long-term dysfunction. Outside of emergencies, care gets sliced into parts. It treats organs, symptoms, and diagnoses in isolation rather than seeing how everything works together. A migraine sends you to neurology. Digestive issues land you at the gastroenterologist. Fatigue? Maybe your endocrinologist takes a look. Each provider stays in their lane, communication is rare, and connection is almost nonexistent.

This fractured perspective is not new. Over 2,000 years ago, Socrates warned, "For this is a great error of our day in the treatment of the human body, *that physicians separate the mind from the body*."[3] He saw what modern medicine continues to miss. Stress reaches far beyond mood. It influences immune function, digestion, hormone signaling, and sleep.

I watched it play out in real time. Every finals week, my body crashed with fatigue, headaches, and sickness as a full-body reaction to emotional overload. Current research has caught up, confirming what many of us have lived. High-pressure environments, especially in medicine and academia, tank immune resilience and keep the body on edge. Up to 90% of all disease is linked to stress because the body remains in survival mode with no clear way out.[4]

The origin of the word "disease" reveals even more. *Dis* means lack or out of balance, and *ease* means comfort or the body's natural state. At its core, disease is a state of imbalance. When the pressure becomes constant, our preferred alignment starts to slip. Rather than asking why that imbalance begins in the first place, the healthcare system moves straight to patches. A symptom shows up. A prescription gets written. Relief becomes the goal, not resolution.

When stress is behind the majority of illness, the most powerful medicine is not going to be found in a prescription pad. It comes from how we eat, move, rest, and reconnect with what our bodies have been asking for all along. Sophia was not the only one paying the price. We are all living in a world where chronic disease has become the default.

THE SOBERING STATISTICS

Today, nearly 74% of American adults and 40% of children are overweight or obese.[5] Chronic conditions like heart disease, diabetes, and Inflammatory Bowel Syndrome (IBS) plague our loved ones more than ever before.

Autoimmune diseases are rising at an alarming rate, increasing by up to 12.5% every year.[6] Nearly half of Americans will face cancer in their lifetimes, meaning in a room of ten friends, at least four will be diagnosed. One in five women is prescribed an antidepressant, while fertility rates are plummeting.[7,8] Since the year 2000, sperm counts have been dropping by 2.3% annually, and infertility rates are rising just as quickly.[9]

We are struggling to maintain a healthy weight, start families, and stay optimistic despite healthcare spending growing every year. According to the CDC, 90% of healthcare costs go toward chronic conditions, all largely preventable through lifestyle changes.[10] With 4.7 billion prescriptions written annually, it is clear our health crisis is not caused by a lack of medication.[11]

The rising rates of disease are not random. They are the consequences of a system built to prioritize treatment over prevention. To understand how we got here, we have to revisit a chapter of medical history that never made it into your textbooks.

THE DARK HISTORY OF MODERN MEDICINE

The turning point in American medicine came in 1910 with the release of the Flexner Report, funded by the Rockefeller Foundation.[12,13] The report declared healthcare must be based on science and tied to universities, dismissing holistic and alternative approaches as "pseudoscience." It established institutions like Johns Hopkins as the gold standard of care, sidelining centuries-old practices based on rhythm, nourishment, and the body's natural intelligence.

On the surface, this shift looked like progress. Breakthroughs in technology, surgical techniques, and pharmaceutical innovation reshaped what medicine could do. Lives were saved, but something essential slipped through the cracks. The body was no longer viewed as a unified system and instead became a set of compartments. As this model took hold, care became symptom-driven, where headaches, fatigue, or weight gain were not traced back to their common roots. They were medicated into silence.

THE RISE OF PHARMA

By the 1960s, the emphasis on symptoms reached new heights with the introduction of the first long-term daily medication: women's birth control.[14] Known as "the pill," it was celebrated as a victory for women's rights, granting autonomy over reproductive health and professional opportunities. While it reduced pregnancies, the pill also birthed a new era of healthcare centered on pharmaceuticals designed for daily, indefinite use.

Drug companies swiftly recognized the immense profitability in chronic conditions. Disease did not need to be cured; it only had to be maintained, which turned long-term management into a business model. Medicine drifted away from restoration and toward symptom control, more interested in quieting the noise than fixing the wiring. It was like silencing a smoke alarm without ever checking for fire.

THE ADDICTION ECONOMY

Around the same time, the U.S. Surgeon General's Report on Smoking and Health confirmed what many had long suspected: smoking is bad for you.[15] Smoking was linked to lung cancer, heart disease, and a host of other life-threatening illnesses. For the tobacco industry, one of the most profitable sectors of the time, this revelation was an existential threat. Faced with declining public trust and plummeting revenue, cigarette companies pivoted.

By the 1980s, the two largest tobacco companies, Philip Morris and R.J. Reynolds, began acquiring food companies. *Why would cigarette companies get involved in food manufacturing?* The answer is simple. Addiction sells.

The same strategies used to hook people on cigarettes were repurposed to engineer ultra-processed foods that were cheap, convenient, and nearly impossible to resist.[16] Foods like neon orange cheese puffs and sugar-packed breakfast cereals were deliberately crafted to hijack taste buds and keep consumers coming back for more.

By the 1990s, aggressive lobbying introduced the now infamous food pyramid, pushing Americans toward a high-carb, high-sugar diet. Refined products took over grocery stores, filling household pantries, including my own. As a child, I reached for the "healthier" choices my thoughtful mother carefully selected, like granola and fruit snacks. We were unaware that what looked nutritious on the outside was silently inflicting harm. It was not until I got sick in adulthood that I began connecting the dots. Ultra-processed foods had been driving inflammation in my body and brain all along. Like most people, I had been misled by clever food marketing that continues to feed the chronic disease epidemic today.

FOOD PYRAMID GUIDE

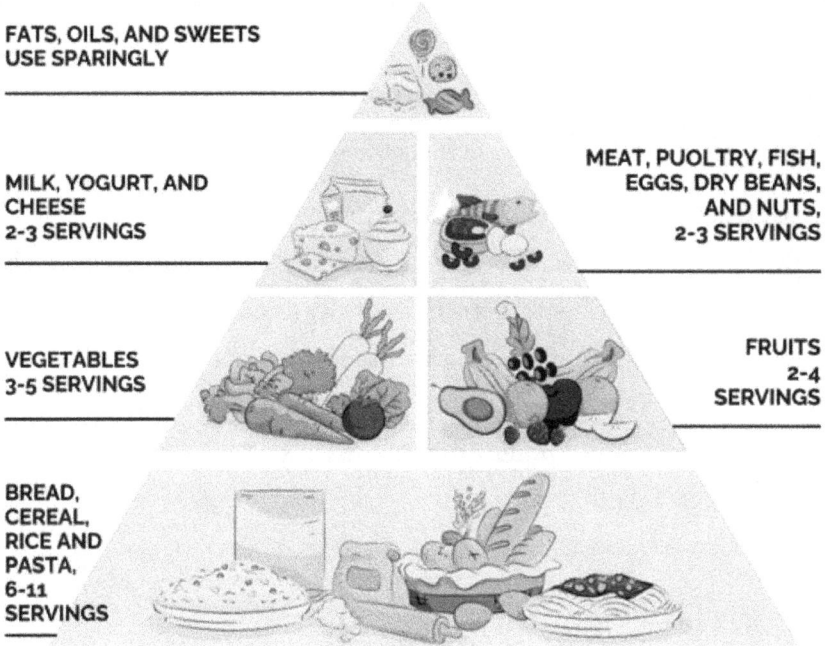

FATS, OILS, AND SWEETS
USE SPARINGLY

MILK, YOGURT, AND
CHEESE
2-3 SERVINGS

MEAT, PUOLTRY, FISH,
EGGS, DRY BEANS,
AND NUTS,
2-3 SERVINGS

VEGETABLES
3-5 SERVINGS

FRUITS
2-4
SERVINGS

BREAD,
CEREAL,
RICE AND
PASTA,
6-11
SERVINGS

THE COST OF QUICK FIXES

The pharmaceutical and food industries worked in tandem, laying the groundwork that fuels the public health crisis we now face. Rather than addressing the root causes, they designed a system propped up by quick fixes:

- If a child struggles to sit still, they are given Adderall.
- If a teen is obese, they are handed weight-loss injections.
- If an adult feels low, they are prescribed an antidepressant.

Instant relief gets handed out like candy while the underlying issues remain untouched. We have drifted far from the natural rhythms that once tethered our health. Days are spent indoors under fluorescent lighting, glued to screens, and snacking on foods our ancestors would not recognize as edible. Conditions that would send wild animals to madness have become our baseline yet, we wonder why we are unwell.

Consider how animals live in harmony with the world as they eat off the land, rest in the sun, and avoid stressors that threaten their safety. I watch my cat sunbathe daily, fully at ease, without need for a meditation app. Humans have lost these instincts and traded them for productivity, convenience, and stimulation. We have uprooted ourselves from the alignment that nature intended and we are paying for it with our health.

THE PATH FORWARD

Blame does not belong here. Most people are not unhealthy because they are lazy. Deep down, we all desire to feel good, clear, and capable. Over time, though, we have been conditioned to fixate on what we can measure, medicate, or mute, while the real issues stay out of sight.

The good news is we are not powerless. Healing begins when we stop viewing our symptoms as problems and instead view them as messengers. We shift from asking *"How do I get rid of this?"* to *"What is my body trying to tell me?"*

I wrote this book because I know what it is like to feel out of sync, chasing worthless solutions, questioning if a foggy, disconnected version of life was my new normal. My healing did not come from a gimmick or a one-size-fits-all plan. It started the moment I stopped fighting my body and finally started understanding it.

Healing is not about rejecting modern medicine. It is about reconnecting to the Earth, to yourself, and to the wisdom your body has carried all along. That intelligence is still there, rooted deeply, just hidden beneath layers of distraction and misinformation.

We are going to dig it up, starting with the core driver behind every decision, sensation, symptom and stress response: your nervous system.

CHAPTER 2

WIRED FOR WELLNESS

"God may forgive your sins, but your nervous system won't."
– Alfred Korzybski

"I've had hormone tests, thyroid exams, and everything else. They all come back normal, and I'm made to feel I'm crazy, so I just stop trying. I'm so depressed because I'm losing hope that I can ever be normal again."

Amelia's message stopped me mid-scroll. It was not just her words, but the weight behind them. The kind of heaviness that builds when your body keeps breaking down with no answers. After two decades of symptoms and second opinions, she was drained in every sense of the word.

DISMISSED AND DISHEARTENED

At 45, Amelia was still trying to piece together what had gone wrong. For over 20 years, she collected symptoms like some people collect coffee mugs. Determination was not her problem. She had consulted every office—neurologists for headaches, gastroenterologists for constipation, fitness trainers for weight loss, and her primary care physician for fatigue.

As I reviewed Amelia's intake forms, I wondered if there was anything she had not tried. Fiber supplements, elimination diets, colonics, and cleansing pills had all been recommended, but none helped long-term. She even underwent exploratory bowel surgery, hoping it might uncover an answer to her digestive drama. It did not.

At their peak, Amelia's headaches were so severe they would rob vision from one eye while leaving her entire right side numb. Medication did not help, and neither did sleep. She regularly clocked 12 to 14 hours a night and still woke up feeling more exhausted than when she went to bed.

Belly fat clung to her midsection like it had signed a lease. No trainer, supplement, or injectable could move it, not even human growth hormone or phentermine. She powered through workouts and relied on coffee and energy drinks, attempting to cut through a brain fog so thick it felt oppressive.

Amelia appeared as the modern American woman in a nutshell: struggling to tone up, dealing with bloating and fatigue, and cycling through medications. Because she was not at immediate risk of hospitalization, doctors brushed off her symptoms as a byproduct of aging. For too long, she almost believed it. Until we met.

ENDING 20 YEARS OF TRIAL AND ERROR

Amelia had tried everything except pausing long enough to question the habits keeping her stuck in survival mode. We started with a lifestyle audit to take an honest look at the patterns training her nervous system to expect chaos.

- **Nutrition:** Amelia's diet centered around convenience. Coffee on an empty stomach fueled her busy mornings, lunch was a *maybe* depending on her workload, and dinner often came late, heavy on the ultra-processed foods because she rarely had the energy to cook.

- **Recovery:** Amelia worked overnight shifts in law enforcement, sometimes for weeks at a time. She often went days without proper sleep and then spent her weekends collapsed on her couch to charge up enough for the next rotation.

- **Light:** She spent most of her time indoors, averaging eight hours a day at screens, long after sundown. She rarely saw natural daylight.

- **Movement:** Outside of a single weekly personal training session, Amelia remained largely sedentary, spending her days in a patrol car or parked at a desk.

- **Toxins:** From personal care products to chemical household cleaners, Amelia's environment was loaded with toxins. Living in polluted Las Vegas, she also drank unfiltered tap water daily.

- **Stress:** Her career required her to manage life-threatening crises while leading a team of officers. As a single woman, she also struggled with loneliness and a lack of meaningful connection in her personal life.

No single habit broke her. The accumulation did, keeping her body in a state of stress. With the full scope of what was contributing to her breakdown, we made sustainable changes. Processed foods were replaced with nutrient-rich meals that supported her metabolism. We built a consistent sleep routine she could stick to, giving her a shot at real recovery. Movement became a non-negotiable, even if it was just a couple of walks around the block. We lightened her toxic burden with cleaner alternatives. Most importantly, we gave her nervous system a reason to exhale.

Six months later, Amelia was a different woman. She could enjoy meals without bloating, sleep without waking up groggy, and live without debilitating headaches. Energy came without caffeine, her weight dropped naturally, and she weaned off all medications. The biggest shift was not physical. Amelia came back to herself with confidence so big she even landed an acting role on a TV show!

Amelia got her life back after spending half her of it chasing symptoms. She was fully present and her shift had nothing to do with a magic pill. It started with regulating her nervous system, the true command center for everything including energy, digestion, and repair. To truly understand her recovery and your own potential, we need to understand how the nervous system operates.

THE NERVOUS SYSTEM MADE SIMPLE

Your nervous system is the root system of your body, coordinating everything you do, including how you move, feel, and respond to the world around you. It has two large branches: the central nervous system (CNS) and the peripheral nervous system (PNS). The CNS includes your brain and spinal cord, while the PNS connects your brain and spinal cord to your muscles, tissues, and organs.

The PNS splits into two key divisions that govern your actions:

- The somatic nervous system, which controls movements you do on purpose, like brushing your teeth or kicking a ball

- The autonomic nervous system, which takes care of processes running in the background, like your heartbeat and digestion.

Dysfunction in the autonomic branches is one of the biggest drivers behind modern symptoms and chronic inflammation.

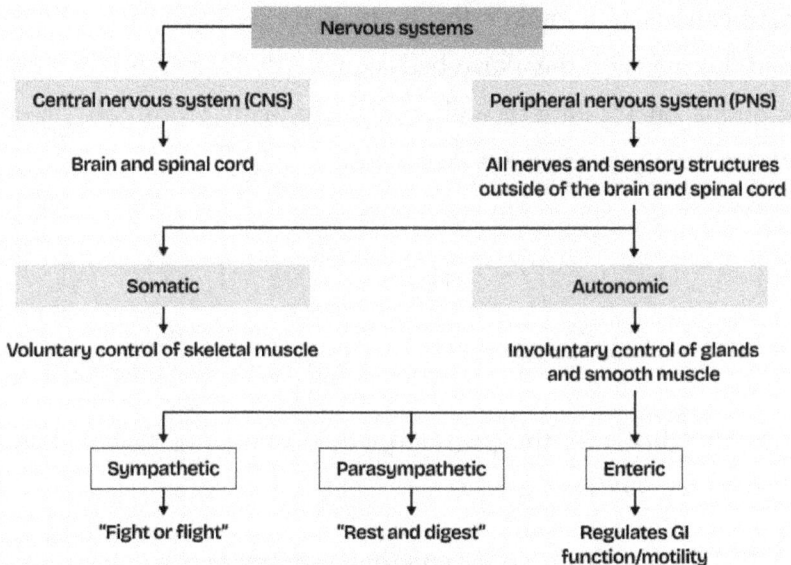

Nervous systems		
Central nervous system (CNS)		**Peripheral nervous system (PNS)**
Brain and spinal cord		All nerves and sensory structures outside of the brain and spinal cord

Somatic	Autonomic	
Voluntary control of skeletal muscle	Involuntary control of glands and smooth muscle	

Sympathetic	Parasympathetic	Enteric
"Fight or flight"	"Rest and digest"	Regulates GI function/motility

FIGHT OR FLIGHT: THE SYMPATHETIC NERVOUS SYSTEM

The sympathetic nervous system is your body's built-in alarm, designed to protect you in times of danger. It triggers the fight-or-flight response whenever a threat is detected.

- Pupils dilate for sharper vision.
- Adrenaline surges through your veins for energy.
- Blood reroutes from digestion to your limbs so you can throw a punch or make a run for it.

This response is brilliant in true emergencies. The problem is most of us are not running to escape wild animals like the cavemen did. Instead, we battle work deadlines, traffic jams, and a constant stream of notifications that makes the body react as if we are still being hunted. Living with the alarm bells constantly blaring is like running your phone on 1% battery with every app open. Eventually, it shuts down whether you are ready or not.

REST AND DIGEST: THE PARASYMPATHETIC NERVOUS SYSTEM

On the flip side, the parasympathetic nervous system handles your recovery mode.

- Your heart rate slows, creating a sense of calm.
- Digestion functions optimally, breaking down food and absorbing nutrients.
- Your muscles relax, allowing the body to recharge.

This system is meant to regulate the chaos, but for many people, it is barely accessible. When stress becomes the norm, relaxation starts to feel like a foreign language you forgot how to speak.

THE STRESS SPECTRUM

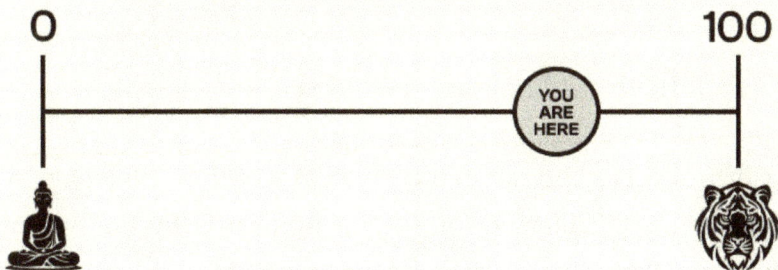

Stress does not flip like a light switch. It moves on a spectrum from zero to 100. At zero, you are like the Buddha, blissed out in a parasympathetic state. At 100, you are in full-blown fight-or-flight, running for your life. Most people are not camped out at either end. They live somewhere around 80, jittery but functional, tired but wired, bracing for the next thing before the current thing even ends.

When the body lives in anticipation of crisis, every system adjusts to survive it. Muscles stay tense, blood sugar swings, hormones spiral, and digestion takes a backseat.

THE STRESS SPECTRUM

0   100

YOU
ARE
HERE

THE GUT-BRAIN CONNECTION

The final branch of the autonomic nervous system is the enteric nervous system, the part that lives in your gut. Often called the "second brain," it oversees digestion, absorption, and elimination. When you are bloated, constipated, or gassy, the root issue often lives here, not in the stomach itself.

My client Francis spent years battling chronic gut issues, eliminating half her food groups, and bouncing between a dozen providers (yes, really). No approach worked because every solution focused on her stomach, not her nervous system.

We flipped the script. Instead of more restrictions, I asked her to stop eliminating and eat what she enjoyed. We focused on creating safety in her body, not fear around food. Within weeks, her bloating vanished, her energy returned, and inflammation started to come down, all without a single supplement. For the first time in years, she stopped pumping out cortisol, the stress hormone driving her symptoms.

CORTISOL IS NOT THE BAD GUY

Cortisol gets a bad rap in the wellness world. Scroll long enough, and you will see it blamed for everything from belly fat to burnout, often followed by ads for adrenal support pills you did not ask for.

Cortisol is not the enemy. It is your body's 911 operator that acts quickly when used correctly. In a true crisis, cortisol keeps you alert, mobilizes energy, and helps you manage pain so you can respond and recover. The problem is not cortisol doing its job. The problem is that your body thinks every email, To-Do, and life curveball is an emergency.

While cortisol is doing its best to keep up, the constant demand drains your reserves and leaves you wondering why you are tired, puffy, and anxious all at once.

THE CHRONIC STRESS HIGHWAY

If you feel like you have been in overdrive or running on fumes, you are likely stuck on what I call the Chronic Stress Highway. It looks like productivity, but leads straight to burnout.

Along the horizontal axis, we have the phases of stress in time. On the vertical axis are cortisol levels, one of the most telling markers of how well your body is coping with stress. As a car on this highway, you are ideally cruising comfortably at 60 miles per hour (mph). You would not want to be stalled out at zero, but you also do not want to be gunning it at 100.

- **Zone 1, the Adaptation Phase**: This is the sweet spot. You are cruising within the speed limit. Your system is regulated and equipped with energy to slow down or speed up without breaking down. Stress enters, and recovery follows.

- **Zone 2, the Acute Phase:** A car unexpectedly tailgates you, so you speed up to 85 mph. Cortisol spikes, and your system shifts into high gear to meet the challenge. If the stressor passes, you can slow back down. If it does not, you are stuck at high speeds for longer than you are designed to sustain, which wears down the tires, and overworks the engine.

- **Zone 3, the Compensatory Phase**: You have been flooring it for too long. Fuel is running low, but your dashboard warning light has not turned on yet, just like your lab results may still look "normal." You feel the wear and tear, so you start reaching for quick-fixes in an attempt to regain control.

- **Zone 4, the Exhaustive Phase**: No matter how hard you press the gas, you are barely moving. Life passes you by as your body runs on fumes, redirecting what little energy it has to survive, which leaves gut health, sex drive, and mental clarity on the side of the road. Most people do not seek help until they reach this final zone. If we want to get off this highway, we need to stop overriding the system before the engine fails altogether.

CHRONIC STRESS HIGHWAY

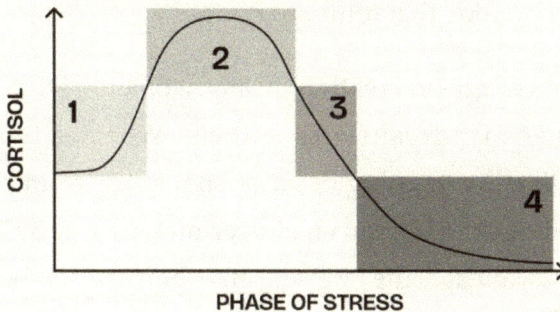

COMMON, BUT NOT NORMAL

Stress does not just live in your head. It weaves through hormones, digestion, and immunity until tension starts to feel like home. Amelia lived there for years. Her labs were "fine," so her symptoms were dismissed as standard. Fatigue, period problems, and weight gain gets blamed on getting older, doing too much, or having bad luck, when in reality they are signs of a body pushed past its limits.

- **Running on Empty:** More than four million Americans suffer from chronic fatigue syndrome, though that number barely scratches the surface. An estimated 90% of cases go undetected.[17,18] Waking up exhausted or relying on coffee to function is not normal. It is a warning the body has been in overdrive for too long.

- **The Cortisol Belly:** Stress-driven weight gain, particularly around the belly, is the body's ancient survival mechanism in action. It stores fat near vital organs to prepare for a famine that never comes, leading to "cortisol belly," or the stubborn last ten pounds that refuse to budge.

- **The Pause on Procreation:** Many women I work with have lost their menstrual cycles entirely. Whether from physical stress like overtraining or emotional stress from overwhelm, the body prioritizes survival over making a baby. It does not want to create life in an environment it perceives as dangerous.

- **Derailing Digestion:** Nearly 40% of Americans report regular bloating, and conditions like IBS and food sensitivities are everywhere.[19] Chronic stress pulls resources from digestion, causing constipation, diarrhea, and imbalances in gut bacteria.

- **Stretched Too Thin:** Stress hijacks the immune system, making you more susceptible to illness. I see this often with professionals who push through projects and periods of intense stress only to get sick the moment they take a break. The body holds on, until it cannot any longer.

Healing starts by reclaiming control, not over everything, but over what is within reach. We are wired for survival, sure, but we are also wired for wellness. When the body feels safe, it remembers how to recover. And that recovery begins with food, the most underestimated medicine we have.

CHAPTER 3

MASTERING YOUR METABOLISM

"When diet is wrong, medicine is of no use.
When diet is correct, medicine is of no need."
– Ayurvedic proverb

Nutrition advice today feels like trying to assemble IKEA furniture without the instructions. It is frustrating, complex, and almost guaranteed to fail. One expert swears cutting carbs is the secret, while another targets fats. Keto says ditch fruit, raw vegan bans anything cooked, and somewhere in the mix, juice cleanses and fat-burning pills promise miracle results. No wonder people feel lost.

Eating was never meant to be this perplexing. Before we had influencers pushing celery juice and almond moms logging calories, people still managed to eat and survive. So, where did we go wrong? A good place to start is with the fact that most doctors receive almost zero training in nutrition. A 2015 study revealed less than 20% of U.S. medical schools required a single nutrition course.[20] They can recite drug interactions in their sleep, but many cannot help you build a plate that prevents, let alone reverses, disease.

Just because the system stalls, we do not have to. Restoring balance will not require eliminating entire macronutrients or using 12-week fad diets with a cult-like dedication. The focus should center on fueling in a way that supports the Hormone Hierarchy.

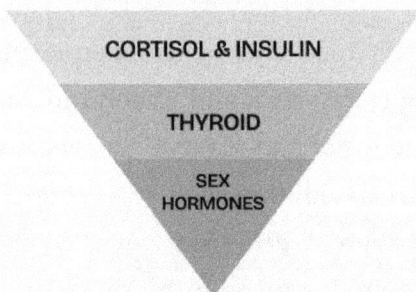

THE HORMONE HIERARCHY

Your hormones operate like an upside-down pyramid, with cortisol and insulin sitting at the top influencing everything downstream. Cortisol handles your stress response. Insulin decides how your body uses and stores energy. When these two are balanced, everything beneath them functions smoothly. When not in equilibrium, the entire system feels it, leading to thyroid disorders, reproductive issues, and weight fluctuations.

Cortisol may get the headlines, but insulin pulls just as many strings, quietly dictating how your body handles fuel.

THE HORMONE HIERARCHY

CORTISOL & INSULIN

THYROID

SEX HORMONES

THE KEY TO YOUR METABOLISM

Insulin's story begins with blood sugar, also called glucose. Glucose is the sugar your body derives from food and its go-to energy source. Glucose is like gasoline for a car. Without it, you are not going anywhere. However, gasoline alone cannot move the car. You need the key to start the engine. Insulin is that key.

Every time you eat, your blood sugar rises. In response, insulin steps in to unlock your cells and escort that sugar inside, where it can be turned into fuel. Problems begin when meals revolve around refined carbs and ultra-processed foods, which spike blood sugar over and over. Eventually, your cells begin to ignore insulin's signals. It is like getting too many texts from an ex. You pay attention at first, but eventually, you just stop responding.

That silence is called insulin resistance and is the gateway to metabolic dysfunction, where the body struggles to manage blood sugar, energy, and fat storage. The insulin key stops working, and glucose builds up in the bloodstream, instead of powering your cells. Nearly 50% of Americans are already there, whether it is labeled as insulin resistance, diabetes, or both.[21,22]

This crisis has quietly become an epidemic. An estimated 93% of U.S. adults show signs of metabolic dysfunction.[23] The damage does not stop at the waistline. It infiltrates every system in the body, including the brain.

MORE THAN WEIGHT MANAGEMENT

When the brain struggles to respond to insulin, the consequences ripple through memory, mood, and mental health. Most people know about type 1 and type 2 diabetes. Fewer have heard of "type 3 diabetes," the term researchers use to describe Alzheimer's disease due to its strong link with insulin resistance in the brain.

Alzheimer's is a progressive neurological disorder that destroys memory, thinking skills, and the ability to carry out basic tasks. It can start subtly, with misplaced keys or forgotten names, before unraveling a person's independence completely. When neurons stop responding to insulin, abnormal proteins build up, damage cells, and lead to cognitive decline. While the connection is unsettling, it can also be empowering. Blood sugar balance gives the brain a fighting chance to reduce the risk of such a devastating diagnosis.

Chronically high insulin also ramps up cortisol, which drags down serotonin. Serotonin is the brain's "happiness hormone," which explains why people with insulin resistance are twice as likely to develop depression.[24]

Mental and metabolic health are inseparable. Blood sugar is the bridge between the two. Once we understand that connection, the next step is learning how to stabilize it.

THE SUGAR BURNERS

Most individuals in the Western world are what I call sugar burners. Their bodies rely almost entirely on glucose, a fast-acting fuel that delivers quick energy. While glucose has its place, it is not meant to work alone. The body is also designed to burn fat and produce ketones, a clean and efficient back up fuel.

Metabolic flexibility is the ideal state. It allows the body to shift between burning sugar for quick bursts and tapping into fat reserves for sustained energy.

You probably know what it feels like to be stuck in sugar-burning mode:

- You ingest something carb-heavy, like a latte and muffin.
- Blood sugar spikes, triggering a flood of insulin to bring it back down.
- Insulin works too well, overcompensating and causing a blood sugar crash.
- You are left feeling tired, cranky, and reaching for more sweet treats.

The cycle repeats all day, every day. A fruit smoothie for breakfast, sandwich at lunch, trail mix for a snack, and pasta for dinner. It seems like a normal way to eat until you are stuck in a cycle of energy crashes, mood swings, and cravings that never seem to let up. Your body was not designed to ride this blood sugar rollercoaster.

WHAT FOOD SHOULD FEEL LIKE

When meals are attuned and metabolism is flexible, you feel it everywhere. Food stops feeling like a guessing game and starts working for you.

- **Stable Energy:** No more hitting a wall at 3 p.m. and reaching for a coffee refill. Instead of needing a post-lunch nap, you power through your workday with focus and clarity.

- **Fewer Cravings:** You are no longer raiding the pantry an hour after breakfast or craving something sweet after every meal. The satisfaction sticks.

- **Improved Mood:** The irritable version of you that shows up when you are hungry? Gone. So is the anxious spiral after a sugar crash.

- **Feeling Lighter:** Instead of bloating or sluggishness, you stay comfortable, without the need to loosen your pants after dinner.

FUELING FOR FITNESS

Tatiana was the woman people turned to when they wanted weight loss results. As a nurse and nutrition coach, she had the credentials, the discipline, and a track record of hundreds of clients who felt like walking success stories. Her own body, however, was not getting the memo. She checked every wellness box: whole foods, quality sleep, and workouts on the calendar. Yet, her energy dragged, and the scale crept up like a personal vendetta. The disconnection shook her confidence. How could she inspire others when she no longer felt like herself?

When we peeled back the layers, the issue was not a lack of effort. It was blood sugar. Her meals were packed with nutrients, but the rhythm and timing worked against her metabolism. Her system had lost its flexibility, stuck in sugar-burning mode with no idea how to switch gears.

We realigned the basics. She learned to build meals that supported stability, not chaos. Tatiana's energy levels surged, inflammation eased, and her body responded by shedding 20 pounds. Her success was rooted in three fundamental nutrition principles:

1. Eat in the right order.
2. Eat at the right time.
3. Eat mindfully.

1. EAT IN THE RIGHT ORDER

Sugar-loaded oatmeal, pancakes, and smoothies have been dubbed the typical American breakfast foods, which spike both blood sugar *and* cortisol, draining your energy reserves well before lunchtime. It is no wonder most people crash by mid-morning.

Research reveals that the sequence in which you eat your macronutrients (carbohydrates, proteins, and fats) has a major impact on how your body processes meals throughout the day. Carbohydrates, like grains, fruits, and legumes, are the body's go-to energy source, but they spike blood sugar the most. Proteins, found in foods like meat, fish, and eggs, cause a much smaller rise. Fats, found in nuts, seeds, and oils, barely budge blood sugar at all. This is why keto diets, which drastically limit carbs, are often praised for stabilizing blood sugar. However, keto is not a long-term solution, nor is it necessary. Your body needs all three macronutrients, just in the right balance.

EFFECT OF MACROS ON BLOOD SUGAR

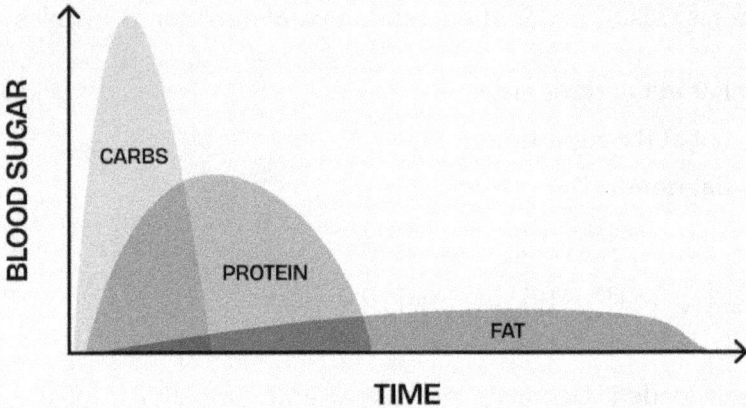

My Golden Rule? *No Naked Carbs.* Carbohydrates should not be eaten alone. That oat milk latte, orange, or granola bar you grab on the way out the door? It is a blood sugar disaster waiting to happen. Instead, think of carbs as the star of the show. They can shine, but only with a strong supporting cast of protein, fat, or fiber.

- **Add Fats:** In a 2014 study, participants ate either plain white rice or white rice with a splash of groundnut oil. Adding fat via the oil reduced their blood sugar spike by nearly 14%.[25] Adding almond butter to a banana has a similar effect.

- **Pair with Protein:** Integrating protein can have an even bigger impact. One study found that mixing protein into a sugary drink reduced the blood sugar response by 23% in men with type 2 diabetes.[26] Another study found that adding 30 grams of protein to a sugary drink blunted the glucose response by 50%. This worked for everyone, whether they were healthy or insulin resistant.[27] If your plate includes a starchy carb like pasta, add a serving of chicken or fish.

- **Don't Forget Fiber:** In a 2010 study, participants sprinkled just five grams of fiber (about a teaspoon) over foods like bread, rice, and granola. Their blood sugar response dropped anywhere from 12 to 45%.[28] You can start with a side salad or steamed veggies before the main course.

HOT DOC WALKS

When meals are heavier in carbohydrates, a brief walk can make a noticeable difference. Active muscles use glucose for fuel, reducing the amount circulating in the bloodstream which eases the burden on insulin.

One study found that adults with type 2 diabetes experienced better blood sugar control by walking for just ten minutes after each meal compared to a single 30-minute walk.[29] Small, consistent movement throughout the day is more effective than one large effort. Consider the Hot Doc Walk a simple prescription for better blood sugar, digestion, and metabolic health.

2. EAT AT THE RIGHT TIME

Timing matters. The same meal can impact your blood sugar differently depending on when you eat it. A Harvard study found that eating later in the day, between 1 p.m. and 9 p.m., led to increased hunger, fat storage, and higher obesity risk compared to eating between 9 a.m. and 5 p.m.[30] The body is primed to process food during daylight hours when energy demands are naturally higher.

Another proven way to support blood sugar is narrowing the eating window through time-restricted feeding (TRF). TRF is not about starvation. It supports your body's natural cycles, improving glucose control, enhancing gut repair, and sharpening brain function. TRF also fosters metabolic flexibility, training your body to switch seamlessly between burning sugar and fat for energy. A 2021 study showed that eating within a ten-hour window stabilized blood sugar levels, improved insulin sensitivity, and even prompted weight loss, all within 12 weeks.[31]

A simple place to start:

- First meal at 8 a.m.
- Last bite by 6 p.m.

This schedule gives your body 14 hours overnight to regulate insulin and shift out of fat storage mode. As blood sugar becomes more stable, many people naturally shorten their window without even trying.

3. EAT MINDFULLY

In our fast-paced world, meals have become another task to squeeze in between meetings, scrolling through social media, or inhaling while watching TV. I have had my fair share of lunches hunched over my laptop in the name of "efficiency." When we eat while distracted or stressed, we keep our body stuck in fight-or-flight mode. Digestion gets downgraded as the nervous system reroutes energy toward survival, leaving food partially broken down.

Most people do not realize digestion does not start in the stomach. It begins in the brain. The moment you see or smell food, your body gets to work releasing salivary enzymes to prepare for what is coming. That mouth-watering feeling when you smell Grandma's cookies is your body's natural way of kicking off digestion.

Eating on autopilot skips this crucial step. Without the brain's initial signals, the stomach may not produce enough enzymes or stomach acid to fully break down food. Even the highest-quality organic meal can fall short as nutrients pass through without getting absorbed. Expensive groceries turn into expensive poop.

Mindful eating does not mean you have to make every meal a fine dining experience. You just need to slow down long enough to let your body and brain work together.

- **Engage Your Senses:** Take a moment to actually notice your meal. Look at its colors, appreciate the textures, and inhale the aroma. Those details cue digestion to get going.

- **Chew Thoroughly:** Aim to chew each bite 30 to 40 times until it is the consistency of applesauce. It might sound excessive at first, but it takes the pressure off your stomach and maximizes nutrient absorption.

- **Be Present:** Drop the devices and take a few deep breaths to shift your body into "rest and digest" mode. A slower pace supports blood sugar balance and even lowers your risk of type 2 diabetes.[32]

One mindful meal per day is enough to remind your body it is safe, supported, and allowed to reset. You are not just getting calories in. You are creating conditions for your body to actually use them.

Now that you know *how* to eat, let's talk about *what* to eat.

CHAPTER 4

FOOD FOR THOUGHT

"The food you eat can be either the safest and most powerful form of medicine or the slowest form of poison."
– Ann Wigmore

WALL-E, the animated movie released in 2008, painted a scary picture of a health crisis disguised as a far-off dystopia. Humans were so dependent on technology, they could barely function on their own as they were confined to spaceships, weighing hundreds of pounds. Floating chairs replaced walking, screens engulfed their attention, and robots catered to their every need.

While *WALL-E* is technically fiction, today's health statistics make it feel eerily close to a documentary. Nearly three in four American adults are overweight, with almost half of children following in their footsteps.[33] The numbers do not come from a script. They reflect a pressing reality demanding our attention.

A CULTURE OF CONVENIENCE

Two generations ago, food was simpler. Our grandparents did

not have to navigate a world dominated by drive-throughs, ultra-processed snacks, and instant meals. Food was prepared at home, families ate together, ingredients did not include a paragraph of additives, and convenience was not mistaken for nutrition.

Today, the opposite is true. Grabbing takeout is easier than cooking. We have also been sold "solutions" to health challenges that focus on restriction rather than nourishment, like fat-free fads, weight loss pills, and prepackaged meal boxes. These mindsets have left us more disconnected from real food than ever before. The diagnoses pile on, and we have lost sight of what eating well should look like.

The impact of this disconnection is not seen only in rising disease rates. It shows up in the gut issues, fatigue, and mood swings we dismiss as "normal." I learned this lesson the hard way.

WHAT NOT TO EAT

"Where's the bathroom?" I whispered to the waiter, trying to sound casual while internally begging for teleportation. It was a first date, and my stomach was spiraling fast. In true 20-something fashion, I had avoided food all day to feel confident in a fitted dress. As someone also newly sober, I skipped the wine list and ordered a non-alcoholic beer to pair with the multi-course dinner as a little reward for sticking to the plan. Big mistake.

Minutes after sipping it, nausea, bloating, and sharp stomach pain took over. I nodded along to my date's stories, pretending to listen while silently calculating the distance to the restroom. By the time appetizers landed, I was lightheaded, irritable, and deeply regretting every decision that brought me to this moment. Turns out, the wheat in that alcohol-free beer was the spark. My gut lit up, my mood tanked, and the entire night went sideways. No second date. No digestible dinner. Just inflammation and an awkward ride home.

That dating disaster drilled home a truth I have never forgotten. Nourishing food supports your energy, clarity, and mood. Inflammatory food hijacks all three. The following are the main offenders doing the most damage while hiding in plain sight.

REFINED GRAINS AND GLUTEN

Refined grains, like white bread and pastries, are stripped of fiber and nutrients during processing. They are left as empty calories that spike blood sugar and crash just as quickly. Many also contain gluten, the protein found in wheat, barley, and rye, which can amplify inflammation and stir up a long list of symptoms:

- **Intestinal Irritation:** Gluten can irritate the lining of the gut, leading to bloating, gas, and cramping. For those with celiac disease, it is even more severe, triggering an immune response that damages the intestines. Even without celiac, gluten sensitivity is real and can cause joint pain, headaches, and even mood swings.

- **Molecular Mimicry:** This one is a bit "science-y," yet intriguing. Gluten's molecular structure looks a lot like certain proteins in your body. For people with autoimmune conditions, this can trick the immune systems into attacking healthy tissues by mistake, leading to more inflammation.

- **Glyphosate Contamination:** In the U.S., wheat and other gluten-containing crops are commonly sprayed with glyphosate, a pesticide linked to cancer, hormone disruption, and kidney issues. This might explain why some people struggle with gluten in the States but have no problem enjoying a slice of pizza or fresh bread while traveling in Europe.

- **Leaky Gut:** Gluten is known to trigger zonulin, a protein that regulates the permeability of your gut lining. Think of zonulin as a doorman in your gut. When zonulin opens the door from your intestines, it allows undigested food particles, toxins, and bacteria to escape into your bloodstream. This sets off a wave of inflammation, known as a "leaky gut." Leaky gut leads to symptoms including acne, eczema, brain fog, food sensitivities, and autoimmune conditions.

IS GLUTEN THE VILLAIN FOR EVERYONE?

Some people tolerate gluten without any issues, and if that is you, it is something to celebrate. For others, especially those dealing with unexplained symptoms, cutting back or removing gluten altogether can be a needle-mover. It is a small shift for a massive improvement in how you feel, like realizing that annoying pebble was actually in your shoe the whole time.

SWAPPING FOR SOURDOUGH

There is a reason some gluten-sensitive folks can comfortably enjoy authentic sourdough bread, and it is not magic. It is old-fashioned science, thanks to fermentation.

Grains like wheat, rice, and seeds were not originally engineered with human digestion in mind. Nature built them to withstand the GI tract long enough to sprout on the other side. Cute, right? This resilience is precisely why grains can cause digestive distress, particularly if your gut is already cranky.

Real sourdough bread, not the supermarket stuff slapped with "sourdough flavoring," transforms gluten through a slow, traditional fermentation process. This breaks down gluten proteins by up to 70%, making sourdough gentler on sensitive systems. While still off-limits for individuals with celiac disease, sourdough can be a solid alternative for those experiencing mild gluten sensitivity.

ULTRA-PROCESSED SEED OILS

Seed oils like canola, soybean and corn sound harmless, yet their origins are more mechanical than culinary. These oils were not born from recipes. They emerged as industrial byproducts intended for machinery, not your pantry.

- **The Industrial Revolution:** In the late 1700s, mechanical presses allowed for mass production of seed oils like flax, sesame, and cottonseed, primarily used to lubricate machines. Cottonseed oil gained popularity as a cheap substitute for whale oil, whose supply was dwindling due to overfishing.[34]

- **The Crisco Craze:** In the early 1990s, Seed oils accounted for only 1% of added fat in the American diet. That changed in 1911 when Procter & Gamble introduced Crisco (hydrogenated cottonseed oil) as the trendy alternative to traditional lard. Marketed as "modern" and "healthy," Crisco transformed an industrial lubricant into a kitchen staple basically overnight.[35]

- **The Big Payoff:** By the 1940s, Procter & Gamble donated $1.7 million (worth $30–$40 million today) to the American Heart Association (AHA), securing the endorsement of seed oils as "heart-healthy" alternatives to animal fats. By the end of the 20th century, seed oils accounted for 85% of added fats in the American diet.[36]

Quantity does not equate to quality. Seed oils are loaded with omega-6 fatty acids, which can create a harmful imbalance when not countered by omega-3s. This disruption ignites chronic inflammation, fueling hormone issues, brain fog, and even cardiovascular disease. The heavy refining, bleaching, and deodorizing necessary to produce these oils also strip them of essential nutrients and antioxidants.

Seed oils are everywhere, tucked away in packaged foods, sauces, and even self-proclaimed "health" products. By ditching the seed oils, you can combat inflammation with stable fats like extra-virgin olive oil, coconut oil, grass-fed butter, and ghee. Your food will taste better, your body will feel clearer, and you will wonder why you ever accepted machinery-grade oils as kitchen essentials.

ADDED SUGARS

Added sugars are the undercover agents of inflammation, sneaking into everything from iced coffees to salad dressings. They bring nothing your body actually needs: no vitamins, no minerals, not even a bit of fiber. They offer quick hits of empty energy, causing a sharp blood sugar spike followed by a predictable crash. Sugary foods, particularly those sweetened with high-fructose corn syrup, did not land in our diets by accident.

- **The Sugar Spin:** In the 1960s, the Sugar Research Foundation paid Harvard scientists to downplay the connection between sugar and heart disease, shifting the blame to fats instead.[37]

- **Low Fat Frenzy:** From the 1980s-90s, fat was stripped from foods and manufacturers pumped sugar to make products palatable. Low-fat yogurt, low-fat cookies, low-fat *everything* flooded the market, yet today we are facing record rates of obesity, diabetes, and metabolic disease.

Sugar's hold is not limited to the waistline. It also hijacks your brain's reward pathways, triggering dopamine, the same pleasure-inducing chemical activated by drugs and alcohol. Over time, just like with alcohol tolerance, you need higher amounts to achieve the initial feel-good rush.

The habit starts earlier than we realize. Remember the candy bowl at the doctor's office or the ice cream celebrations for good grades?

Those moments quietly teach your brain to link sugar with comfort, reward, and happiness, hardwiring dependencies that linger into adult years.

Taking just one month away from added sugars can recharge your energy, sharpen mental clarity, and quiet the constant urge for sweets. You may even rediscover the natural sweetness of whole foods. Approach it as an experiment, not a punishment. Begin gently by scanning labels and replacing packaged sweets with naturally satisfying options like fresh fruit. Once you experience life beyond the sugar fog, you might not want to go back.

FUNCTIONAL FOOD

When Leona reached out, she was worn out from years of battling hormonal acne along her cheeks and chin. The painful breakouts had carved deeper scars than those visible on her face. They chipped away at her self-confidence and sense of emotional stability. She had tried every expensive skincare routine, countless facials, and a pharmacy's worth of medications. Each time she thought she was making headway, another flare-up emerged, pulling her back into the frustrating cycle.

Through targeted functional testing, we identified exactly what was fueling Leona's stubborn acne: elevated androgen hormones intensified by a diet heavy in inflammatory foods. Androgens overstimulated her skin's oil glands, clogging pores and driving breakouts. Processed snacks, sugary drinks, and low-quality dairy worsened the hormonal imbalances. Leona's acne was not just skin deep. It was a direct manifestation of metabolic dysfunction.

Armed with clarity, Leona moved away from the topical treatments and turned inward. Packaged snacks were swapped for fresh produce. Sugary sodas were replaced with refreshing lemon water, making hydration more enjoyable. Healthy fats like avocado and olive oil made their way into her meals, nourishing her skin and bringing her hormones back into harmony.

The results did not take long to surface. In just weeks, redness and inflammation subsided. Over the months, her skin cleared entirely. For the first time in years, Leona felt comfortable going makeup-free, a milestone she thought was out of reach. Leona's glow-up was a reminder that fuel is feedback. When you give your body the right inputs, it radiates.

WHAT TO EAT

Food is both fuel and biochemistry. Every bite either stabilizes your system or sends it spinning. Here are the essentials to build a strong plate:

1. MICRONUTRIENTS: THE MISSING MEDICINE

Micronutrients may needed in small amounts, but their impact is enormous. They fuel energy production, regulate biological processes, and fight oxidative stress, the cellular damage caused by free radicals.

Free radicals act like tiny sparks flying inside your body. Left unchecked, they cause wear and tear and accelerate aging. Micronutrients are your fire extinguishers, neutralizing the sparks before they cause damage. Eating antioxidant-rich foods like berries, leafy greens, and green tea serve as the body's built-in firemen to put out the flame before it spreads.

MICRONUTRIENTS CHEAT SHEET

Vitamin D

- **Why It Matters:** Dubbed the "sunshine vitamin," it supports your bones, mood, and immunity. A deficiency can leave you tired, prone to illness, and mentally flat.

- **Sources:** Fatty fish like salmon and mackerel, egg yolks, and 15–20 minutes of sunlight daily.

Magnesium

- **Why It Matters:** Your body's multitasker, involved in over 300 critical functions, including digestion, nerve signaling, and restful sleep.

- **Sources:** Spinach, kale, nuts, seeds, avocados, and quality dark chocolate at 70% cacao or higher.

Zinc

- **Why It Matters:** Essential for hormones, wound healing, and clear skin. It is especially important during cold and flu season.

- **Sources:** Pumpkin seeds, shellfish, lentils, and chickpeas.

B Vitamins

- **Why It Matters:** Your personal battery-pack, converting meals into usable energy, stabilizing mood, and sharpening brain function.

- **Sources:** Eggs, grass-fed meats, leafy greens, and nutritional yeast.

Selenium

- **Why It Matters:** A critical player in thyroid health, metabolism, hair growth, and antioxidant defense.

- **Sources:** Brazil nuts, seafood, beef liver, and shiitake mushrooms.

Vitamin E

- **Why It Matters:** Another antioxidant, enhances insulin signaling, and supports the immune system.

- **Sources:** Sunflower seeds, almonds, avocados, spinach, and sweet potatoes.

2. PHYTONUTRIENTS: NATURE'S PROTECTIVE COMPOUNDS

Plants do not have claws, fangs, or pepper spray. Their defense system comes in the form of phytonutrients, tiny chemical bodyguards that do a lot more than just keep bugs away. In your body, these compounds cool inflammation, boost detox, and act like armor for your cells in a world full of stressors.

- **Polyphenols**: Found in colorful foods like berries, green tea, and dark chocolate, these compounds are protectors for your gut. Red polyphenols, like those in raspberries, pomegranates, and cranberries, help strengthen your gut lining, reducing symptoms like bloating and food sensitivities.

- **Sulforaphane**: Abundant in cruciferous vegetables like broccoli and kale, this compound aids the liver in detoxifying harmful substances and supports hormone balance, particularly for estrogen. Consider adding broccoli sprouts to your meals, as they pack up to 100x more sulforaphane than regular broccoli.

- **Flavonoids**: Found in citrus fruits, onions, and parsley, flavonoids are overflowing with cardioprotective compounds. They fight inflammation, protect blood vessels, and promote circulation, which is critical since heart disease remains the leading cause of death in the U.S.

60

3. PROTEIN: THE BUILDING BLOCKS FOR LIFE

Protein is not reserved for bodybuilders. It is foundational for everyone to build muscle, repair hair, create hormones, and support a strong immune system.

- Animal proteins like pasture-raised eggs, grass-fed meat, and wild-caught fish are considered "complete" proteins because they contain all nine essential amino acids.

- Plant-based proteins like beans, lentils, and tofu are valuable, but also lack one or more amino acids. If you are vegetarian or vegan, combining sources (like rice and beans) can help fill gaps.

When choosing protein, quality is king. Grass-fed, organic, and pasture-raised options not only taste better but also contain more nutrients and fewer inflammatory compounds than conventional choices.

4. FAT: MANDATORY FUEL

Fat's reputation has been dragged through every diet trend, but your body cannot function without it. Fat helps build hormones, cushions your nerves, and wraps every cell in a cozy little jacket.

- **Omega-3s:** Found in walnuts, chia seeds, leafy greens, and fatty fish like salmon, omega-3 fats are anti-inflammatory and important for brain health. If you have had a foggy brain or struggled with focus, you may be low on omega-3s.

- **Omega-6s:** Although necessary in moderation, omega-6 fats are overrepresented in the modern diet. The typical American diet has a ratio of omega-6 to omega-3 of around 20:1. The ideal ratio is closer to 4:1, which reduces the risk of inflammation for everything from asthma to autoimmune disease.[38]

5. FIBER: YOUR GUT'S PREBIOTIC PERSONAL TRAINER

Fiber is not just for your grandparents. It acts as your gut's personal trainer keeping digestion efficient, well-fed and moving smoothly. Fiber plays a crucial role as a prebiotic fueling the beneficial gut bacteria that support immunity.

Nearly 70% of your immune system lives in your gut. Refined carbs are stripped of fiber and weaken the white blood cells that battle infections. Consuming just one sugar-loaded soda can suppress immune function by 50% for hours.[39]

To keep your gut strong, focus on prebiotic-rich fibers from foods like berries, apples, garlic, onion, lentils, green bananas and ground flaxseeds. You will build an army of good bacteria, reinforcing your body's natural defenses.

6. FERMENTED FRIENDS: PRO AND POSTBIOTICS

Your gut is deeply connected to mood and mental clarity, producing the majority of serotonin, your "happiness hormone." When gut bacteria are out of balance, harmful strains take over. This disrupts serotonin production, raising inflammation and increasing risk for anxiety, depression, and even autism spectrum disorders.[40]

One of the best ways to restore gut equilibrium is by regularly eating fermented foods. If your gut microbiome acts as a garden, fiber is the fertilizer feeding the good gut bacteria already present. Fermented foods introduce healing postbiotics and new, beneficial bacteria via probiotics, as if planting fresh seeds.

Rather than relying on probiotic supplements, which are often ineffective, choose naturally fermented foods like yogurt, kefir, sauerkraut, and miso.

THE LABEL LIES

Food labels are like legal fine print, loaded with loopholes, hidden surprises, and words people do not understand. If you have ever found yourself watching hours of Bobby Parrish's Costco hauls on YouTube just to decode what is actually healthy, welcome to the club.

A simple guideline to follow: if you cannot pronounce it, you probably should not put it in your mouth. The healthiest foods have short, recognizable ingredient lists made up of items you would comfortably stock in your kitchen. Ingredients appear in order of quantity, so the first few dominate the product. If your great-grandmother would not recognize it as food, your body probably will not either.

That said, not all red-flag ingredients are hard to pronounce. Some are hiding in plain sight under simpler names.

Harmful Additives and Preservatives

Many processed foods contain additives designed to extend shelf life, improve texture, or enhance color. While these compounds serve a commercial purpose, they often come with negative effects on gut health, hormones, and inflammation. Some of the most concerning include:

- **Artificial Colors** (Red 40, Yellow 5, Blue 1): Used to make foods look more appealing. These dyes have been banned in countries outside of the U.S. as they are linked to hyperactivity and behavioral issues, especially in children.[41]

- **Carrageenan:** A thickener found in dairy alternatives and ultra-processed foods that contributes to gut dysbiosis, bloating, and chronic gut inflammation, including Inflammatory Bowel Disease.[42]

- **MSG (Monosodium Glutamate):** A common flavor enhancer in packaged snacks, soups, and fast food that can cause headaches, dizziness, and overstimulation of the nervous system.[43]

- **Aspartame & Acesulfame Potassium**: Artificial sweeteners often found in diet sodas, sugar-free gum, and low-calorie snacks. Studies link them to potential metabolic disruptions, increased insulin resistance, and neurological symptoms.[44,45]

Conventional, Organic and Other Certifications

Even if an ingredient list appears "clean," quality and sourcing matter, farming practices, pesticide use, and food certifications provide deeper context into what you are really eating:

- **Conventional Foods:** Typical grocery items grown with synthetic pesticides, herbicides, and fertilizers. Industrial farming depletes minerals so while these foods may seem harmless, they come at a cost to both your health and the environment.

- **USDA Organic:** Grown without synthetic pesticides and fertilizers, though they can still use natural pesticides. Organic is a better choice than conventional, but not always perfect.

- **Pasture-Raised:** The gold standard for animal products. Animals roam outdoors, enjoy fresh air, sunlight, and a natural diet, resulting in meat and eggs richer in nutrients like omega 3s. Picture yourself confined indoors all day versus freely exploring outside. Quality of life translates into quality of food.

- **Regenerative Organic Certified:** A rising movement focused on repairing soil health. Over the last century, industrial farming has stripped the soil of nutrients,

> making today's produce far less nourishing than what our ancestors enjoyed. Regenerative methods rebuild nutrient density and reduce environmental damage.
>
> - **GMO Foods:** Genetically modified organisms (GMOs) are altered in labs for pest resistance or higher crop yields. While debates continue over their safety, legitimate concerns exist regarding their long-term health impact. When possible, steer toward non-GMO choices.

Each meal is an opportunity to nourish your body or deplete it. Small upgrades like swapping canola oil for olive oil or adding variety to your plate may seem minor, yet they add up powerfully over time. Prioritizing quality foods may feel more costly upfront, but chronic illness will cost far more in the long run. Good food is like insurance against a lifetime of medical bills and misery.

Food is foundational, but no amount of clean eating will undo the damage of improper recovery.

CHAPTER 5

LIVING IN SYNC

"Rest is a radical act of self-love in
a world that rewards exhaustion."
– Adrienne Maree Brown

At 23, I was held together by adrenaline and sheer persistence. I would drag myself out of bed at 3:30 a.m. for work, rush to anatomy class by 8 a.m., and end with hours of studying late into the night. Most days, I was lucky to squeeze in five hours of sleep. Evenings blurred together as I stared at my notes, begging my overactive mind to shut off. It never truly did.

Back then, I wore my exhaustion like an unspoken badge of honor. Graduate school demanded I had, and I was all in, even if that meant running myself into the ground. In hindsight, this mindset was not exclusive to my doctoral degree. It was a consistent pattern, starting in college with late-night study binges that often gave way to even later nights out with friends. Once I entered the workforce, the cycle worsened. My relentless "go" mode was fueled by the need to prove myself, to "do it all" for my career, my family, and my expectations.

Ask anyone how they are doing, and the word "busy" is bound to surface. We have turned exhaustion into a status symbol, as if being overwhelmed equals worthiness or success. What no one tells you is that years of burning the candle at both ends does not build resilience. It erodes your energy, focus, and ultimately, your longevity.

You could be eating nutritious foods, smashing your workouts, and spending a fortune on the best supplements on the market, but without proper sleep, you are sabotaging it all.

SLEEP DEBT: THE PRICE WE PAY

Sleep deprivation does not just chip away at health. It steals lives. Every year, over 6000 fatal car crashes in the U.S. are caused by drowsy driving.[46] Thousands of preventable tragedies occur because people are too tired to function. Even more alarming is that pulling an all-nighter impairs judgment, as much as a blood alcohol level of 0.1%, well past the legal driving limit. Running on empty dulls your focus and makes you dangerous.

The damage extends beyond the road. Sleep-deprived workers make more mistakes, take more sick days, and suffer more injuries. Workplace accidents tied to insomnia drain over $31 billion annually, and the broader toll of poor sleep costs the U.S. economy $411 billion every year.[47,48] That includes everything from missed deadlines to catastrophic errors, and it is not limited to office buildings. More than 55% of nurses, our frontline workers, report struggling with insomnia.[49] If the people tasked with saving lives are barely functioning, what does that mean for the rest of us?

THE ULTIMATE RECHARGE

In today's hustle-heavy culture, sleep is the first thing we sacrifice and the last thing we respect. Yet, it remains one of the most powerful tools we have to restore health.

1. Sleep Resets Your Brain

Sleep acts as your brain's overnight cleaning crew and productivity manager. During REM sleep (rapid eye movement), your brain is not idle. It is meticulously organizing the information you processed throughout the day. During this time, ideas are connected, creativity is ignited, and problem-solving improves. A good night's sleep can leave you waking up with solutions to issues that felt impossible the day before.

Now imagine skipping that reset. Without quality sleep, your brain gets cluttered with mental trash. You wake up foggy, sluggish, and struggle to pay attention. Just like your smartphone, your brain needs a full charge to work at its peak.

2. Sleep Keeps You Sane

Everything feels ten times harder after a sleepless night. The amygdala, your brain's emotional control center, becomes hyperactive on low sleep, making you more reactive and anxious. Minor inconveniences like spilling your coffee or missing a turn feel like the end of the world. At the same time, your prefrontal cortex, the rational part of your brain, taps out. You are running on emotional overdrive with little ability to put things into perspective. Quality sleep leaves you calmer, more grounded, and far less likely to spiral over a lukewarm latte.

3. Sleep Balances Your Hormones

When sleep falls apart, your hormones follow. Melatonin, the body's sleep signal, plays a bigger role than most realize. It is essential for regulating rest, but also acts as a potent antioxidant, lowers inflammation, and even protects against certain cancers.

Melatonin does not work alone. Cortisol, thyroid hormones, testosterone, and even human growth hormone (HGH) are all dependent on quality recovery to do their jobs. HGH, the so-called "fountain of youth" hormone, is released primarily during deep sleep. It drives muscle repair and fat metabolism. Testosterone, critical for strength, bone density, and libido in both men and women, is also produced while you sleep. Miss a few solid nights, and testosterone levels can drop by up to 15%, impairing your performance and motivation.[50]

If you are working hard in the gym but neglecting sleep, you are stalling your progress before it even starts.

4. Sleep Bolsters Your Immune System

Your immune system does not work only when you are sick. It is constantly on guard, scanning for threats and eliminating potential invaders. Sleep gives it the upper hand.

During deep sleep, your body produces cytokines, specialized proteins that fight off infections and inflammation. Without enough rest, cytokine production drops, and immune cells become sluggish, leaving you more prone to colds, viruses, and chronic illness.

There is a reason "get some rest" is still the go-to advice when you are under the weather. The body heals faster when it sleeps, and recovery starts by giving it the time to do so.

5. Sleep Curbs Cravings and Aids Fat Loss

After a late night, your breakfast cravings shift fast. That veggie omelet does not stand a chance next to syrup-covered carbs and anything that comes in a paper bag. This is not emotional eating. It is hormonal havoc driven by leptin and ghrelin.

- Leptin signals satiety, telling your brain, "Hey, we're full. Put the fork down."
- Grehlin triggers hunger, yelling, "Feed me now!"

When sleep takes a hit, so do these signals. Ghrelin ramps up, leptin fades, and you are more likely to overeat foods you would not normally choose. Poor sleep also disrupts blood sugar. In one study, healthy men who slept only four hours a night for six days developed pre-diabetic blood sugar levels.[51]

Sleep deprivation also elevates cortisol levels, signaling the body to store more fat, especially around the midsection. You cannot out-exercise poor sleep. If fat loss is your goal, sleep is not optional.

THE OTHER TWO-THIRDS OF THE EQUATION

When people think about rest, they picture sleep, those sacred eight hours each night. However, true renewal does not stop at bedtime. The other two-thirds of the restoration equation plays out during the day, shaped by our relationship with light.

I will clear one thing up early: I am not anti-technology. I will not ask you to toss your phone into a canyon and live by candlelight. We live in an expansive era where we can stay connected across continents, run businesses from our couches, and even meet "the one" online. The problem is not progress. It is the pace. While our devices have evolved at lightning speed, our biology is still stuck in the Stone Age. This mismatch is disrupting hormones, trashing sleep, and tanking metabolic health on a massive scale.

THE ISSUE WITH ARTIFICIAL LIGHT

Childhood obesity rates began to climb sharply in the 1980s, the same decade the home computer became a household staple. As kids spent more time indoors, movement declined, and exposure to artificial light surged. Televisions, fluorescent bulbs, and eventually smartphones extended waking hours and disrupted circadian rhythms that had guided human biology for thousands of years. What began as entertainment slowly rewired the way we sleep, eat, and live.

By 2016, research linked excess artificial light exposure to 70% of overweight and obesity risk factors.[52] The connection goes far beyond reduced outdoor playtime. Blue light exposure at the wrong times primes the body for fat storage and long-term weight gain. To fully understand how screens have quietly shaped our health, we need to look at their impact on the body's natural rhythms.

Trends in obesity among children and adolescents ages 2-19 years, by age: United States, 1963-1965 through 2017-2018

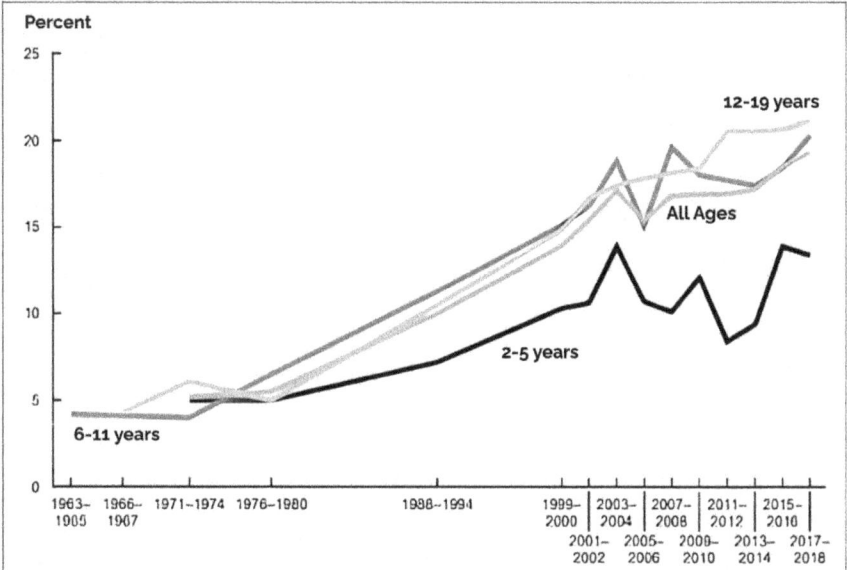

Percent

[A line chart titled with percent on the y-axis ranging from 0 to 25, and year ranges on the x-axis from 1963-1965 through 2017-2018. Lines labeled "12-19 years", "All Ages", "2-5 years", and "6-11 years" trend generally upward over time.]

(Source:[53])

THE CIRCADIAN RHYTHM

Your circadian rhythm is a 24-hour internal clock run by a tiny brain region called the suprachiasmatic nucleus. Despite the complicated name, its job is simple: keep your body's systems in sync. In an ideal world, your circadian rhythm would run like clockwork:

- **Morning:** Cortisol peaks, fueling energy and focus.
- **Evening:** Melatonin rises to help you relax and recover overnight.

Cortisol and melatonin operate like a seesaw. When one rises, the other falls. That rhythm sets the tone for everything from alertness to recovery, keeping your body on schedule. For most of human history, time itself was the guide. Sunrise signaled movement, and sunset meant rest.

Then, blue light barged in and blurred the lines. Emitted from phones, laptops, TVs, and LED bulbs, blue light sends the wrong message at the wrong time. Your brain interprets it as midday sun, even if it is 10 p.m. on your couch. The false signal spikes cortisol, shuts down melatonin, which results in restless sleep, slower recovery, and a higher risk of chronic disease. And we are soaking it in from morning to midnight.

SCROLLING OURSELVES SICK

The average U.S. adult spends over seven hours a day on their phone, not including laptop or TV time. Teenagers are even worse, racking up eight and a half hours daily, not counting classwork. Social media alone eats up an average of two hours and 23 minutes per day.[54] That is an entire month of every year spent scrolling through reels, TikToks, and status updates. Over a lifetime, it translates to nearly a decade spent inside apps instead of real life. Imagine what you could build, become, or create if you took even half that time back.

All that screen time steals your attention and also rewires your nervous system. The CDC reports that teenagers who spend four or more hours per day on screens are significantly more likely to experience anxiety and depression than those with less exposure.[55] This is not a generational overreaction. It is a physiological response.

The more time we spend glued to screens, the more we block the signals our bodies need to regulate mood, focus, hunger, and rest. Often, it takes a break to realize how overstimulated we have actually been. Time in nature does not just feel good. It resets the nervous system in ways scrolling never could. You do not need to move to the mountains to reverse the damage. You can start syncing with your biological clock in real time.

HOW TO SYNC YOUR NATURAL RHYTHM

1. Limit Artificial Light

The easiest, most effective way to improve your circadian rhythm is by mastering your light environment. No fancy technology required.

- **Use Red Bulbs in the Evening:** Red light has the least impact on melatonin, making it the ideal choice for spaces where you unwind.

- **Black Out the Bedroom:** Even tiny amounts of light can disrupt melatonin. Invest in blackout curtains, an eye mask, or both. My own sleep setup includes earplugs, a white noise machine, mouth tape (yes, it is a thing), and complete darkness.

- **Wear Blue Light Blocking Glasses:** Clear lenses claiming to limit blue light barely filter out the high-energy wavelengths that disrupt melatonin. Amber or orange-tinted glasses block the specific range of blue light that tells your brain it is daytime. Wearing them two hours before bed helps keep your sleep hormones on track.

- **Unplug:** The simplest fix is often the best one. Shut off the TV, dim the lights, put your phone on airplane mode, and give your body permission to wind down naturally.

2. View Sunlight

Humans are diurnal by design, wired for activity during the day and restoration at night. That rhythm depends on light, specifically photons passing through the retina and signaling the brain what time it is. Without that cue, your body starts guessing, and it is usually wrong.

Morning sunlight acts as your biological anchor. It signals cortisol to rise for energy, boosts serotonin to improve mood, and cues melatonin production later that night. Missing this window can disrupt your internal clock, leaving your body out of sync.

I like to get outside within an hour of waking and spend at least ten minutes in natural light. On cloudy days, I would aim for twenty. No sunglasses, no windows, just your eyes and the sky. Even when the sun is not shining, daylight is still powerful enough to reset your internal clock and get your systems online.

3. Get Rooted in Data

Start tracking your sleep to improve it. I use an Oura Ring in airplane mode, but you do not have to invest in an elaborate tracker to benefit. Utilize a sleep journal to jot down when you go to bed, when you wake up, and how you feel throughout the day. Once you have done this for a week or so, you will have enough data to identify patterns and fine-tune these three key metrics:

- **Quantity:** The total number of hours you sleep each night. The sweet spot for most is seven to nine. If you are constantly clocking less than seven hours, your body is not getting enough time to recharge.

- **Quality:** Quantity is important, but not all sleep is created equal. Sleep quality comes down to what is happening while you are snoozing:

  - **Latency:** How long it takes you to fall asleep. The ideal range is 10 to 20 minutes. If you are out the second your head hits the pillow, you might be running on empty, a sign of overtiredness or chronic sleep deprivation. If it takes you longer than 20 minutes, factors like stress or caffeine might be interfering.
  - **REM and Deep Sleep:** REM is essential for memory, learning, and emotional processing, while deep sleep is where physical repair, hormone release, and immune support happen. Aim for about 90 minutes of each per night.

- **Consistency:** Your body loves routine. Going to bed and waking up at the same time, yes, even on weekends, stabilizes your circadian rhythm. I am a big advocate for setting a bedtime alarm. We always set alarms to awaken, but how often do we remind ourselves when it is time to wind down?

SHIFT WORK DOESN'T HAVE TO BREAK YOU

Circadian rhythm thrives on consistency. So what happens when your schedule is a mess? For shift workers like my client Jake, sleep felt like a lost cause. Even through relentless nights and zero routine, we built a system that worked with his biology, not against it.

Jake worked as a government nuclear operations specialist, logging grueling 12-hour night shifts for up to two weeks straight. After a day or two to recover, he was thrown right back into high-stress conditions that pushed his nervous system past its limits.

By the time he reached out, his exhaustion had spiraled into something far more concerning. He was struggling with severe mood swings, unexplained skin rashes, and chronic digestive issues. Comprehensive functional testing confirmed what we suspected: his immune system was depleted, and his adrenal glands were on the brink of burnout.

Jake's job was actively working against his circadian rhythm, so our strategy focused on stabilizing his internal clock with a schedule he could not escape.

- **Set the Clock:** Jake followed a consistent sleep-wake schedule every day, including his days off. No sleeping in, no catch-up naps. Predictability became medicine.

- **Utilize the Light:** Darkness signaled rest. We blacked out his bedroom post-shift, ditching screens and minimizing stimulation. Bright light therapy helped simulate morning sun during his waking hours to anchor his alertness and improve his energy curve.

Within three months, his body caught up. His energy returned, his skin cleared, and for the first time in decades, he felt like himself again. As he put it, "I feel amazing. I get great sleep. I have way more energy, and I don't feel my age anymore. I actually feel like I did when

I was in the military." Jake's success is a testament to the body's ability to heal. Even the most challenging schedules can be managed with the right approach.

However, not every one has a night shift to blame. Maybe you have cut the screens, gotten your sunlight, nailed the routine and you still find yourself staring at the ceiling at 2 a.m.

THE INSOMNIA EPIDEMIC

Insomnia is more common than most realize, affecting one in four women and one in five men.[56] If you find yourself struggling to fall or stay asleep, consider these often-overlooked rest wreckers:

Rest Wrecker 1: Poor Meal Timing

Meal timing is one of the sneakiest disruptors of quality sleep, and convenience culture has not done us any favors. Too many people skip meals during the day, only to overeat at night. Instead of easing into repair, you are rerouting energy to your gut.

On the other hand, going to bed hungry can be just as disruptive, triggering hunger cues that wake you up mid-sleep cycle. The golden zone is wrapping up your final meal two to three hours before bed. That window allows your body time to process food, stabilize blood sugar, and settle into a restorative rhythm.

A NOTE ON THE "SLEEPY GIRL MOCKTAIL"

Social media has a new favorite sleep hack: the "Sleepy Girl Mocktail." Recipes vary, but most include tart cherry juice (for its natural melatonin), magnesium powder, sparkling water, and a squeeze of citrus.

I appreciate the concept of creating a bedtime ritual, however, tart cherry juice contains considerable amounts of natural sugar, even the unsweetened versions. Drinking the mocktail mix right before bed can spike blood sugar, leading to a midnight crash that wakes you up.

If you want to try it, follow the No Naked Carbs rule. Pair your cherry juice with a protein or fat, like a handful of nuts, to buffer the blood sugar spike. If you want a safer bet, skip the sugar altogether and opt for a high quality magnesium supplement or calming tea like chamomile instead.

Rest Wrecker 2: Alcohol

That nightly glass of wine might feel like a comforting way to unwind, but alcohol is more of a sleep thief than a sleep aid. It acts as a sedative, helping you fall asleep quickly. Yet it suppresses REM, the stage your brain relies on for emotional processing and cognitive repair.

When REM is disrupted, sleep becomes fragmented. Even if you do not remember waking up, those micro-interruptions prevent your body from reaching the deeper stages needed for hormone regulation, muscle repair, and immune strength. What feels like relaxation on the surface is often quietly stealing the recovery your body needs most.

Rest Wrecker 3: Caffeine

Caffeine is a common crutch, the go-to for staying sharp, powering through deadlines, and shaking off exhaustion. However, if you are tossing and turning at night, your afternoon coffee habit could be the culprit.

Caffeine's half-life is about five hours, meaning that if you have a cappuccino at 3 p.m., half the caffeine is still in your system by 8 p.m. Depending on your metabolism, it can linger for eight to ten hours or longer, subtly sabotaging your ability to wind down.

I suggest you set a caffeine curfew. Most people benefit from cutting off caffeine at least ten hours before bed. If your goal is to be asleep by 10 p.m., your last cup of coffee should be no later than noon.

Rest Wrecker 4: Liver Burden

Your liver is your body's detox powerhouse, filtering out toxins and metabolizing everything you have been exposed to throughout the day.

According to Traditional Chinese Medicine (TCM), the liver is most active between 1 and 3 a.m. If you consistently wake up during those areas, it might be a signal from your liver indicating that it is under strain or struggling to keep up its workload. There are deeper imbalances that deserve attention, which you can read about in Chapter 8.

THE 10-3-2-1 RULE: YOUR BLUEPRINT FOR BETTER SLEEP

My favorite framework to optimize your evenings to wake up energized and restored is the 10-3-2-1 Rule.

- **10 hours before bed**: Cut off caffeine. This allows your body time to fully metabolize it.

- **3 hours before bed**: Stop eating. By giving your digestive system time to slow down, your body can focus on repair instead of processing a heavy meal.

- **2 hours before bed:** Limit water intake. Reducing late-night hydration helps prevent disruptive wakeups for bathroom trips.

- **1 hour before bed:** Power down screens. Reducing blue light exposure supports melatonin.

The way you sleep dictates the way you live. Your day starts the night prior. Without deep, restorative rest, your body is uprooted, stuck in survival mode, and your hormones pay the price.

CHAPTER 6

LET'S TALK ABOUT SEX (HORMONES)

*"If you didn't come from a healthy family, make sure
a healthy family comes from you."*
– Unknown

You would think with all the fertility apps, hormone tests, and prenatal supplements flooding the market, we would be in the middle of a baby boom. Instead, we are in a fertility-free fall. Over the last 50 years, men's sperm counts have dropped by more than 50%, testosterone levels are sliding lower each decade, and infertility now affects 1 in 9 women.[57,58] Conditions like polycystic ovary syndrome (PCOS), the leading cause of infertility, have gone from overlooked to almost expected, impacting over five million women in the U.S. alone.[59]

Reproductive health is more than making babies. It is a mirror of deeper hormonal, metabolic, and nervous system functions. When fertility falters, it is usually a signal that something foundational has fallen out of rhythm.

INFERTILITY IS EVERYONE'S ISSUE

Despite how it is often portrayed, fertility challenges are not exclusive to women. Both partners play a role, and today, both are increasingly affected. The World Health Organization defines infertility as the inability to conceive after twelve months of unprotected sex, a reality that now impacts one in six individuals worldwide.[60] Picture six of your closest friends or family members. Statistically, conceiving will be a heartbreaking challenge for one of you.

It takes two to make a baby, yet male reproductive health is rarely part of the conversation. Sperm quality, motility, and hormonal integrity are just as critical. When men are left out of the picture, timelines stretch, answers stay buried, and blame often shifts unfairly. The focus shifts to quick-fix solutions like birth control, hormone replacements, and surgeries without ever addressing the underlying disconnection.

NO BABIES, JUST BURNOUT

Reproduction was not designed to compete with inboxes, exhaustion, or the expectation to have it all figured out by 30. Fertility has been reduced to a box to check, not a rhythm to honor. A Morgan Stanley study predicts that by 2030, 45% of women ages 25-44 in the U.S. will be single and likely childless.[61] The obsession with productivity has made it tougher to build relationships, create stability, and prioritize sexual health. Career demands, financial burdens, and constant stress have pushed parenthood further down the list, only for many to discover their bodies are operating on a different timeline.

We are facing a paradox. More people require fertility support, yet few are tending to reproductive health, often until it is too late. This does not mean everyone must have children. However, something is clearly wrong in a society where nearly half the population struggles to conceive, waits too long, or opts out because they are overwhelmed or worn thin. The real concern is not just how to make a baby, but why we have created an environment where so many physically, financially, or emotionally cannot.

Fertility is not just a medical outcome. It is a reflection of capacity. When the body does not feel safe, it downshifts reproduction to protect its resources.

THE CORTISOL CONNECTION

Infertility often starts with stress, a force so woven into daily life that most people stop noticing it. Deadlines pile up, bills creep in, workouts blur into overtraining, and the grind never lets up. Your body clocks it all as a threat and shifts into survival mode.

When your brain senses danger, making a baby drops to the bottom of the priority list. Your body does not want to bring a child into an environment it deems is unsafe. The goal becomes survival, not conception. To meet the demands of stress, the body diverts resources toward cortisol production, pulling from the same hormone pool needed for reproduction.

All sex hormones, estrogen, progesterone, and testosterone, share a common precursor: pregnenolone, often referred to as the "mother hormone." Pregnenolone is like a teacher managing its hormonal students. If cortisol starts having a meltdown and throwing chairs, pregnenolone shifts all its attention to quiet the noise. Meanwhile, the calmer students, your sex hormones, lose the support they need to stay on track.

Over time, that trade-off drains the resources, keeping cycles regular, ovulation steady, and libido alive. Testosterone tapers, progesterone disappears, and reproductive health takes a back seat while your nervous system tries to keep the wheels from falling off.

Just as a chaotic classroom can find peace with the right teacher, hormones can recalibrate with the right guidance.

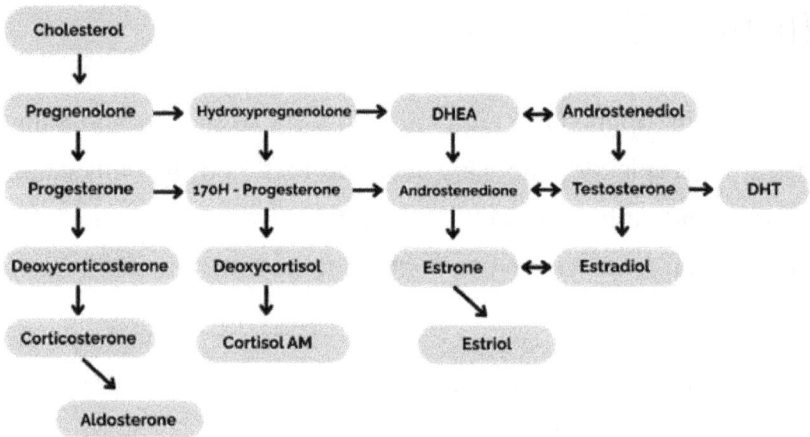

NO PERIOD, NO PROBLEM

Hormones can take a hit, but even the most resilient system has its limit. Nancy had passed it. At just 23 years old, her period had been missing for over a year. A history of hormonal birth control, rigorous bodybuilding, and the emotional aftershock of her father's sudden passing left her body locked in survival mode. Ovarian surgery added another layer of stress, stripping away what little hormonal stability she had left.

As a health coach, Nancy knew the textbook answers. Yet, no amount of knowledge could outpace the reality she was living. Her metabolism slowed, bloating was constant, and her energy was so low that simple tasks like washing dishes felt insurmountable. Lab results painted a full hormonal picture: sky-high cortisol and bottomed out sex hormones. Her hormone panel read more like someone twice her age and she felt completely disconnected from her young body.

She did not need another protocol or stricter meal plan. Her body was drowning in cortisol and desperate for relief. As we settled her nervous system, the hormone chaos started to clear. Within just three months, Nancy's period returned like clockwork. Her digestion calmed, energy rebounded, and her resilience resurfaced. Her story reminds us that hormone dysfunction is not permanent. It is a signal. When you love your body, it will love you back.

Hormonal breakdowns are everywhere, and not because we are fragile. They are rooted in an education gap we have carried since childhood.

YOUR SEX ED CLASS SUCKED

When I was a teen, the only lesson I absorbed regarding sex was to not have it, or I would get pregnant. That was it. Nothing about hormones or what a healthy period should look or feel like. There was certainly no guidance on how to spot red flags. Even saying the word "tampon" felt taboo.

By the time I turned 16, I was handed birth control before I was sexually active, as if that were some kind of rite of passage. No one mentioned the side effects. No one asked about my symptoms. That gap in hormonal literacy set me up for a decade of chronic symptoms.

I count myself as one of the lucky ones. I got out early and managed to undo the damage before I traveled down the path millions take: $40,000 sunk into in vitro fertilization (IVF), undergoing painful procedures, and feeling powerless in their own bodies.[62,63]

In fact, only 18 states require sex education to be medically accurate, leaving kids and young adults clueless about their own biology.[64] Of course hormones feel confusing. You deserve better intel than fear-based lectures and outdated diagrams. I am going to break it down clearly, simply, and in a way that actually sticks.

MEET YOUR HORMONE DREAM TEAM

Men and women share the same core hormones, just in different amounts. Your hormones operate like a championship team. Each player has a critical role, and when they work together, everything runs smoothly. But if one player slacks off or steals the spotlight, the whole system starts to unravel.

LUTEINIZING HORMONE (LH): THE COACH

LH calls the plays, making sure everything stays on schedule. It signals the testicles to produce testosterone in men and triggers ovulation in women. Without LH leading the team, the game never even starts.

FOLLICLE-STIMULATING HORMONE (FSH): THE TRAINER

FSH works behind the scenes, getting players like sperm and eggs ready to perform. It matures sperm in men and preps eggs for ovulation in women. Without it, the team has no viable players.

TESTOSTERONE: THE STAR ATHLETE

Every winning team has a game-changer, the one who sets the pace, delivers the power, and pushes past limits. Testosterone is the Michael Jordan, fueling muscle growth, stamina, and motivation in both men and women. Similar to an athlete who has lost their edge, testosterone levels are steadily declining, throwing performance and recovery off track.

- **In Men:** Men rely on testosterone to dominate the game, but levels are dropping by 2.3% annually.[65] A man in his 20s today will have significantly lower testosterone in his 50s than previous generations, leading to poor performance at his work, the gym, and in the bedroom. A star player cannot carry the team if they are out of fuel.

- **In Women:** Though women require far less testosterone, it is still essential for strength, drive, and sexual vitality. A natural mid-cycle boost explains why some women feel more energized and confident during ovulation. When testosterone runs low, symptoms like muscle weakness, weight gain, and sluggish metabolism creep in, often mistaken for stress or aging.

Signs and Symptoms of Imbalanced Testosterone	
High Testosterone	**Low Testosterone**
Acne	Low libido
Irritability	Impaired sexual function
Lack of impulse control	Decreased muscle mass & strength
Hair loss on scalp	Dry, thinning hair & skin
Hair growth on face, chin, chest (women)	Hot flashes
Insomnia	Depression
Ovarian cysts	Poor concentration & memory
High blood pressure	Fatigue
Weight gain	Weight gain

WHY TESTOSTERONE LEVELS TANK

Low testosterone is not a fluke. It is a direct result of lifestyle, stress, and environmental exposures. Here is what can throw the MVP off its game:

- **Lack of Healthy Fats:** Hormones are built from cholesterol. Cut too many fats, and your body struggles to keep its key players in action.

- **Xenoestrogens:** Found in pesticides, plastics, and personal care products, these estrogen-mimicking chemicals block LH, the signal that tells your body to produce testosterone.

- **Excess Body Fat:** Fat cells convert testosterone into estrogen through aromatization, tipping the hormonal balance in the wrong direction.

- **Toxic Mold Exposure:** Mold lowers MSH, a hormone that helps regulate the pituitary gland, the command center for testosterone production.

- **Certain Medications:** Painkillers, statins, beta-blockers, SSRIs, hair loss meds, Spironolactone, and some antifungals are all known to suppress testosterone.

- **Chronic Stress:** When cortisol dominates the field, testosterone gets benched. In survival mode, your body prioritizes stress management over hormone production.

TOO MUCH ROCKET FUEL?

High testosterone might sound like a good thing, but too much can throw off the entire team. Here is what can send levels well past their sweet spot:

- **Over-Supplementation:** Many young men turn to testosterone boosters for muscle growth or performance, but pushing levels too high can backfire, leading to hormonal chaos and even long-term infertility.

- **Poor Diet:** Diets high in refined carbs and sugars fuel insulin resistance, which reduces sex hormone-binding globulin (SHBG). With less SHBG to regulate it, free testosterone levels skyrocket, a common trigger for PCOS. The result is irregular cycles, excess facial or body hair, acne, and ovulation issues.

- **Chronic Stress:** Just like low testosterone, excessive levels can stem from prolonged stress. The adrenal glands produce small amounts of testosterone, but when stress overloads the system, both cortisol and testosterone spike, a double-whammy disaster.

ESTROGEN: THE TEAM CAPTAIN

If testosterone is the MVP, then estrogen is the captain who ensures the team moves as one. Estrogen orchestrates movement, coordinates plays, and influences everything from brain function to metabolism.

- **In Women**: Dubbed the "Queen Bee" of hormones, estrogen is the backbone of female health. It protects bones, supports heart function, sharpens cognition, and regulates the menstrual cycle. When regulated, it keeps the body agile and adaptable. But when estrogen goes rogue, either too high or too low, it can trigger PMS symptoms and metabolic slowdowns.

- **In Men**: Men need just the right amount of estrogen to keep testosterone in check, maintain vascular health, and support cognitive function. Too much can lead to fat retention, low libido, and mood imbalances. Too little is a recipe for stiff joints, brain fog, and even heart problems.

A strong team cannot win without strategy and precision, and estrogen is the playmaker, ensuring everything runs smoothly. Even in the hormone world, the team needs both strength and coordination.

Signs and Symptoms of Imbalanced Estrogen	
High Estrogen	**Low Estrogen**
PMS symptoms	Hot flashes
Water retention & bloating	Night sweats
Tender breasts	Painful intercourse
Mood swings	UTIs
Headaches & brain fog	Headaches & brain fog
Low libido	Depression & anxiety
Sleep disturbances	Joint pain
Histamine intolerance	Fatigue
Endometriosis, gallbladder issues, cysts	Weight gain

QUEEN BEE OFF HER GAME?

Estrogen may be the playmaker, but when she is off her game, the whole team feels it. Here is what can throw the Queen Bee off:

- **Lack of Healthy Fats:** Just like testosterone, estrogen needs cholesterol as a raw material.

- **Hormonal Birth Control (HBC):** Birth control overrides natural hormone production, shutting down ovulation, tricking the brain into thinking estrogen is covered, and masking PMS symptoms. HBC use results in a withdrawal bleed that is not a true period and a depletion of key nutrients like magnesium and B vitamins that are essential for hormone balance. Worse, women who use birth control for over a decade have up to a 38% risk of developing breast cancer, an estrogen-sensitive cancer.[66] The risk was shown to remain for at least five years after discontinuation of HBC.

- **Gluten Sensitivity:** Research links gluten-related issues to missing periods, reduced ovarian reserve, and infertility, suggesting that underlying inflammation may interfere with estrogen production.

- **And, of course, Chronic Stress.** Stress steals the spotlight and hormone production gets sidelined.

ESTROGEN DOMINANT?

Too much estrogen can be just as disruptive as too little. From mood swings to painful periods, the Queen Bee needs the right amount of control. Too much power, and the game gets messy. Here is what can cause estrogen overload:

- **Low Fiber Intake:** Estrogen gets escorted out of the body through stool. Without enough fiber, particularly soluble fiber, excess estrogen can be reabsorbed in the body instead of eliminated.
- **Sluggish Liver:** The liver acts as the cleanup crew, breaking down and clearing out used hormones. When liver detox pathways get overwhelmed, whether from stress, poor diet, or toxins, estrogen lingers too long.
- **Overaromatization:** This process converts androgens, like testosterone, into estrogen. Aromatization takes place primarily in fat cells, so the more fat tissue you have, the more this conversion occurs, raising estrogen levels further.
- **Caffeine and Sugar:** Caffeine can spike estrogen levels, leading to irritability, anxiety, and more intense menstrual cramps. Meanwhile, refined sugar depletes magnesium and drives insulin resistance, which further stimulates aromatase, leading to even more estrogen.
- **Alcohol:** Even moderate drinking can temporarily raise estrogen levels, placing extra strain on hormones, especially during perimenopause and menopause when the system is already recalibrating.

PROGESTERONE: THE DEFENSIVE LINE

Progesterone is the rock-solid defense that keeps the team stable and protected. It acts as a buffer, preventing energy crashes, hormone swings, and metabolic chaos.

- **In Women:** Progesterone is the steady foundation that keeps cycles regular, moods stable, and inflammation in check. It also promotes deep sleep, supports brain health, and protects against estrogen dominance.

- **In Men:** While men produce much less progesterone, it plays a key defensive role by balancing testosterone, supporting sleep quality, and keeping stress hormones in check. Without enough, cortisol can take over, leading to higher estrogen, sluggish metabolism, and poor recovery.

Signs and Symptoms of Low Progesterone
Hot flashes
Facial hair growth
Hair loss (scalp)
PMS
Irregular or missing cycles
Osteoporosis
Sleep disturbances
Anxiety and depression

Progesterone Benched?

When progesterone is sidelined, estrogen overpowers, testosterone wavers, and the system loses homeostasis. Some reasons why progesterone might be out of the game include:

- **Lack of Healthy Fats:** Like other sex hormones, progesterone production requires healthy fats.

- **Hormonal Birth Control:** Just like in estrogen, HBC stops ovulation, meaning no natural progesterone is produced.

- **You Guessed It, Chronic Stress:** High cortisol output steals the ball, forcing your body to pay less attention to progesterone.

High progesterone is far less common, but can result from over-supplementation, infections, or pregnancy (which is a win if you are trying to conceive!).

WHY MEN SPRINT AND WOMEN FLOW

Same hormones, different timelines. Men are sprinting and women are pacing a marathon. One system thrives on consistency. The other thrives on attunement. When either one is ignored, the cost is steep leading to chronic dysfunction.

LET'S TALK ABOUT SEX (HORMONES)

DAILY PEAKS: THE MALE HORMONE CYCLE

Testosterone in men follows a 24-hour circadian rhythm. Levels rise and fall predictably across the day:

- **Morning Surge:** Testosterone peaks early, boosting mental sharpness, physical stamina, and the well-known physiological response upon waking. With high energy and focus, it is the perfect time to tackle tough projects, push through intense workouts or enjoy intimacy.

- **Midday Dip:** Levels begin to taper slightly, but focus and motivation hold steady. Men are more at ease compared to the morning but still driven and upbeat. It is optimal for collaboration and strategic thinking.

- **Evening Low:** As testosterone continues to drop, the body naturally shifts into recovery mode. Energy softens, signaling it is time to slow down, relax, and reconnect.

While men recharge on a 24-hour loop, women operate on a more layered cycle that spans weeks, not hours.

TWO CLOCKS, ONE BODY: THE FEMALE HORMONE CYCLE

Women move through both the circadian rhythm and an additional biological cycle called the infradian rhythm. The infradian rhythm ranges between 23-35 days, governing the menstrual cycle, influencing energy, metabolism, and emotional bandwidth across four distinct phases:

- **Follicular Phase (7–10 Days):** Estrogen rises post-period, sparking creativity, motivation, and resilience. This is the best time for personal growth and taking on new challenges.

- **Ovulatory Phase (3–4 Days):** Estrogen and testosterone peak together, amplifying confidence, libido, and social energy. This phase amplifies confidence and makes it ideal for networking, collaboration, and intimacy.

- **Luteal Phase (10–14 Days):** If pregnancy does not occur, progesterone takes over, calming the body. Energy naturally slows, lending itself to deep focus and setting boundaries. PMS symptoms may surface here, especially if hormones are unbalanced.

- **Menstrual Phase (3–7 Days):** Hormones hit their lowest levels, making rest, reflection, and self-care non-negotiable. Overexerting yourself during this time can backfire.

Forcing your way through every phase as if your body stays the same can carry real consequences, including an increased risk for PCOS, endometriosis, and chronic fatigue syndrome. Mental health takes a hit too, with women twice as likely to experience anxiety or depression.

Fighting your biology is a losing game. The real win comes from aligning with it. For men, that means riding the wave of daily testosterone peaks. For women, it is learning how to flow with a cycle that was never meant to stay static.

ACHIEVING HORMONAL HARMONY

Whether your body operates on a daily circuit or a monthly rhythm, hormone health relies on strategy. Performance can shift with proper nutrition, minimizing toxin exposure, and a regulated nervous system.

1. Balance Your Blood Sugar

When your hormones feel like they are throwing a tantrum for no reason, blood sugar might be the instigator. Insulin resistance does not only mess with energy. It flips the whole Hormonal Hierarchy. In men, it pushes testosterone toward estrogen conversion, leading to lower sex drive, higher fat storage, and chronic disease like type 2 diabetes. In women, it worsens irregular cycles and conditions like PCOS.

As discussed in Chapter 3, meal timing matters. Research shows consolidating meals into an eight-hour window improves insulin sensitivity, aids weight loss, and enhances menstrual regularity in women with PCOS.[67] Hormones love rhythm. Give them consistency, and they will stop acting like toddlers.

2. Reduce Endocrine Disruptors

Plastic containers, synthetic skincare, chemical-coated produce, none of it is harmless background noise. These disruptors mimic hormones, block receptors, and confuse your body's messaging system. The fix does not involve living off-grid. In Chapter 8, we will cover how to make a few smarter swaps in your kitchen, bathroom, and shopping cart to support hormones.

3. Calm Your Nervous System

Chronic cortisol surges suppress testosterone, disrupt ovulation, and push the body into "not safe to reproduce" mode. Until your nervous system feels secure, your hormones stay in a panic. Chapter 9 outlines proactive strategies to regulate stress for better hormone function.

Once hormones are steady, timing becomes everything. Understanding when fertility peaks unlocks a smarter, more intuitive approach to both connection and conception.

UNDERSTANDING THE FERTILITY WINDOW

Hormonal rhythms offer a natural blueprint for men and women to align their intimacy and family planning goals. Still, most of us were taught that pregnancy is always just one slip-up away. Birth control became the default, and many grew up believing that any unprotected sex equals a baby. The truth is conception can only occur within a small fertility window, roughly six days each month:

- **The five days leading up to ovulation:** Since sperm can live in the reproductive tract for up to five days, waiting for an egg to arrive.

- **The day of ovulation:** An egg is released and ready for fertilization.

During this window, many women experience a natural surge in testosterone, boosting energy and libido. It is no coincidence that nature syncs peak fertility with peak connection.

BEYOND BIRTH CONTROL

When you understand the fertile window, you stop outsourcing your health and start making confident, informed decisions. Natural cycle tracking offers an intelligent way to plan, prevent, or prepare on your terms:

1. **Observe Cervical Mucus:** Before ovulation, cervical mucus is scant, sticky, or creamy. As estrogen rises, it becomes clear, slippery, and stretchy, like egg whites. This is a key sign that ovulation is approaching. After ovulation, progesterone thickens and dries up cervical mucus, making conception unlikely.

2. **Predict Ovulation:** Ovulation Predictor Kits (OPKs) measure the surge in LH that occurs 24-48 hours before ovulation. A positive result indicates ovulation is likely to occur within the next 1-2 days.

3. **Track Basal Body Temperature (BBT):** BBT is your resting body temperature, measured right when you wake up, before moving or getting out of bed. It can be taken orally, vaginally, or rectally. Just stick to the same method for consistency. Tracking BBT helps identify when ovulation has occurred:

   • Before ovulation, BBT is lower, typically 97–97.7°F.

   • After ovulation, progesterone causes a 0.5–1°F spike, which remains elevated until a woman's next cycle.

   • If you note three or more days of sustained higher temps, ovulation has happened.

- When BBT stays elevated for 18 days or more, it could be an early sign of pregnancy and time to grab a test!

While BBT tracking is a powerful tool, certain factors can impact its reliability, including lack of rest, illness, stress, medications, environmental changes, travel, and alcohol. BBT is most accurate when one has had at least three uninterrupted hours of sleep.

Hormone health includes fertility, feeling grounded, and in sync with what your body needs. When you are rooted in your rhythm, energy, metabolism, and connection flow naturally. Once you learn to read the hormonal signals, you train, rest, and move in ways that builds you back up.

CHAPTER 7

MOVEMENT IS MEDICINE

"We don't stop playing because we grow old;
we grow old because we stop playing."
– George Bernard Shaw

Before I built a health practice, I built playlists and taught high-intensity group fitness classes like my rent depended on it. Technically, it did. For six years, I worked at a popular franchise with thousands of studios worldwide, priding itself on maximizing calorie burn. The energy in the room was contagious, but the conversations I had with members after workouts told a different story.

Women would approach me, frustrated, asking why all their hard work was not translating into results. They would say, "I'm here multiple times a week, and I eat clean, but nothing's changing." Some had even been told by their doctors that weight gain was just a part of aging.

What they did not realize was that the one-hour workout they were squeezing into their busy schedules, while valuable, was not enough on its own.

STOP BEING A GYM TOURIST

As a society, we are simply not moving enough. Despite the U.S. having more gyms than any other country, 76% of children and adults do not meet the recommended physical activity guidelines.[68,69] Meanwhile, in the world's Blue Zones (the regions with the highest concentration of folks living to at least 100), people are not grinding out hours in a fitness center. Instead, they integrate movement into their daily routines: walking to the market, tending to gardens, or engaging in mindful activities like yoga.

The cost of a sedentary lifestyle is astronomical. Physical inactivity adds up to $117 billion each year in healthcare expenses, yet one of the most simple and effective solutions is often overlooked: walking.[70]

Walking is not "just walking." It is a catalyst for health. Just 30 minutes a day, five times a week can significantly lower the risk of heart disease.[71] Walking also:

- Supports weight management
- Stabilizes blood sugar
- Reduces symptoms of depression and anxiety
- Lowers the risk of osteoporosis and arthritis
- Increases lifespan

Taking 8,000 steps per day drops your risk of death by 51% compared to 4,000 steps. If you bump up to 12,000 steps a day, the risk decreases by an incredible 65%. Yet, the average American only takes between 3,000 and 4,000 steps per day.[72]

We need to move with the intention and consistency of athletes, not the sporadic enthusiasm of gym tourists. A single intense workout a week, no matter how taxing, will not make up for ten hours of sitting. Movement is like showering. You cannot take one power wash on Monday and expect to stay fresh come Friday.

While movement builds strength and endurance, it also supports one of your body's most intricate balancing acts in blood sugar.

THE BLOOD SUGAR DANCE

By now, you know your body runs on glucose. Every bite you take gets broken down into sugar and sent into the bloodstream to fuel everything from your early-morning workout to late-night brain dumps. That fuel needs somewhere to go and when your muscles are inactive, glucose has no outlet. So your body does what it is designed to do and stores the excess as fat and waits for instructions.

Movement changes the equation. Whether you are walking the dog, squatting under a barbell, or dragging your toddler through Target, your muscles pull glucose from the blood to keep up. Once immediate fuel runs out, your body switches to use stored fat. Over time, this promotes metabolic flexibility and supports sustainable weight management.

You do not have to live at the gym for it to count. Cleaning the house, taking the stairs, or walking kids to school all add up.

MUSCLE: THE LONGEVITY ORGAN

Muscle is an essential driver of longevity. Dr. Gabrielle Lyon calls it "the world's longevity organ" for good reason.[73] It is more metabolically active than fat, burning more calories at rest. Muscle tissue also creates more insulin receptors, or "keys," which means your body can keep your blood sugar levels steady more effectively. The benefits of strong, healthy muscle include:

- Consistent energy
- Enhanced performance
- A body primed to build even more muscle

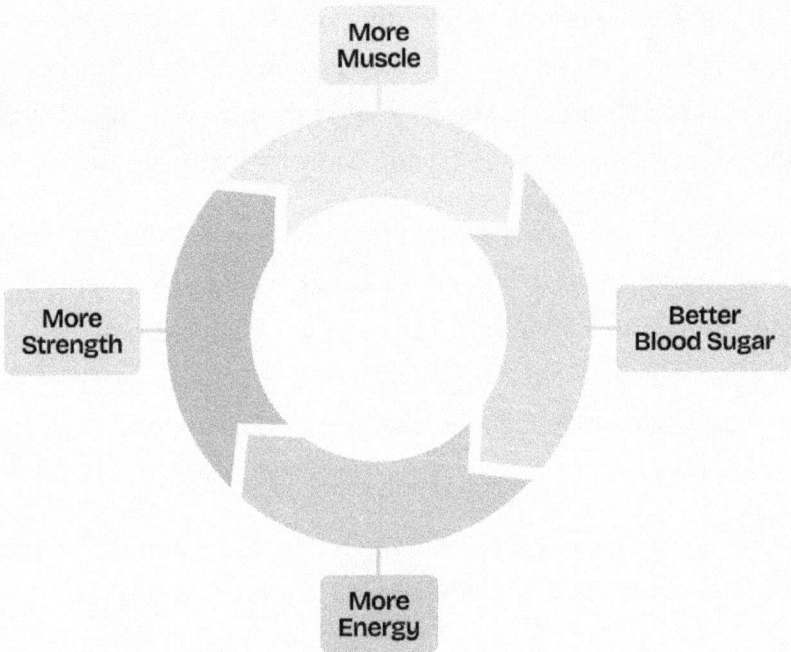

More Muscle

More Strength

Better Blood Sugar

More Energy

THE HOTEL HOUSEKEEPER STUDY: WHY PERCEPTION MATTERS

Sometimes, how we think about movement matters just as much as the movement itself. In one study, researchers divided hotel housekeepers into two groups.[74] One group was told their daily tasks, like vacuuming and scrubbing, counted as exercise. The other group was told nothing.

Four weeks later, the first group lost weight, reduced their blood pressure, had better body fat percentages, and had lower BMIs simply by believing they were exercising. The uninformed group had no change. When you perceive movement as beneficial, anything can be "exercise." Perception is powerful. So is pressure. While movement can heal, overtraining can do the opposite.

THE DARK SIDE OF FITNESS

I learned the hard way that more exercise does not always lead to better results. Sometimes, it means a full-blown system failure. During my first bodybuilding season, I reached 107 pounds at 5'5" with body fat so low I looked like a walking anatomy chart. It was perfect for the stage but unsustainable for survival. I was lifting weights five days a week, doing two hours of cardio per day, and running on pure passion.

After my first competition, my body was screaming for rest. Instead of allowing it to recover, I pushed through a second show two weeks later. That is when the wheels came off. I developed mast cell activation syndrome, a condition where immune cells overreact. My

ROOTED

skin erupted in relentless, full-body itching that lasted six weeks straight. I could not sleep. I could hardly think.

Then came the rebound. Within six months, I gained back 30 pounds without binge eating, which is a common struggle in the bodybuilding world. Some of the weight was necessary, but much of it felt like my body had hit the panic button. The following year, I attempted to lose some of the extra body fat, but it only made things worse. I gained another 13 pounds in just four weeks. My cortisol had tanked, and my nervous system went into full-on fight-or-flight. The spiral ended in not one, but two autoimmune diagnoses, and the kind of wake-up call you do not ignore twice. If I were to attempt training again without wrecking my health, I had to consider my hormones.

EXERCISE LIKE A GIRL

Overtraining affects everyone, but women are especially vulnerable. Unlike men, whose hormones reset every day, cycling women operate on a second, less predictable clock tied to menstruation (see Chapter 6). Energy, metabolism, and recovery shift throughout the month, meaning women's bodies are not designed to always be operating at high intensity.

In the follicular phase, the week or so after a period, estrogen and testosterone rise which supports fat loss and muscle growth. Strength gains feel easier, crushing a HIIT class feels good, and motivation is easier to source.

The luteal phase is a different story. As the body prepares for a potential pregnancy, metabolism kicks up, burning an extra 300 calories per day. That does not mean it is time to double down on workouts. Recovery slows, cortisol sensitivity increases, and the body becomes less efficient at handling high stress. A study published in *Sports Medicine* showed endurance declines more rapidly during this phase.[75,76] Push too hard, and women will get the diminishing returns of more fat storage, more muscle breakdown, and a nervous system that is on edge.

CYCLE-SYNCHING WOMEN'S WORKOUTS

Syncing workouts with your cycle is not about doing less. It is about being strategic with the physiological shifts across the month to enhance performance.

- **Turn Up the Heat:** The follicular phase is primetime for progress. Energy levels are higher, and a surge in hormones supports fat-burning and muscle-building. Take advantage of this window by sprinting, trying CrossFit, or using heavier weights. Personal bests tend to land here for a reason.

- **Dial It Back to Build Smarter:** Once progesterone takes the lead in the luteal phase, your system needs a different kind of support. Swap high-intensity sessions for yoga, Pilates, or moderate resistance training. Incorporate rest days and listen to internal cues. Pushing too hard can elevate cortisol, leading to symptoms in and out of the gym.

For morning workout lovers, working out on an empty stomach may feel like a high in the follicular phase. However, fasted workouts in the luteal phase may leave women feeling fatigued and stressed. A small pre-workout snack during their luteal phase can stabilize blood sugar and keep your body from mistaking exercise for a threat.

The menstrual cycle is not a roadblock to fitness. It is a roadmap. When women align their workouts to their biology, they unlock strength, speed, and real results.

ENERGY IN MOTION

Exercise does more than build strength. It is one of the fastest ways to reset your mood and rewire your mindset. The word "emotion" comes from the Latin root meaning "to move out," reinforcing what many of us have felt firsthand. Movement is medicine when mental weight sets in.

When anxiety, frustration, or heavy emotions take hold, movement works like a pressure release valve for the nervous system. It clears mental clutter and brings the body back to center. Science backs this up. Physical activity boosts neurotransmitters that influence how we feel, think, and function:

- **Dopamine:** The brain's built-in motivator. It sharpens focus, drives momentum, and delivers the post-workout satisfaction or reward of crossing off a to-do list.

- **Serotonin:** The emotional stabilizer. Serotonin keeps us calm, grounded, and reduces anxiety.

- **Endorphins:** Nature's painkillers. Endorphins are often associated with the "runner's high" that helps ease stress, leaving us feeling refreshed and uplifted.

You do not need marathon workouts to feel the shift. Instead, focus on integrating small bursts of activity to help you move through and process big feelings.

MINIMUM MOVEMENT GOALS

If you are not training for the Olympics, you do not need to live at the gym. What your body craves is consistency. Movement supports both healing and health when it is part of daily life, not something squeezed in after a weekend of brunch and regret. These minimums create a steady foundation your system can rely on.

- **8,000 Steps Per Day:** No need to chase an arbitrary 10,000-step rule. Research shows that 8,000 steps daily are enough to reduce disease risk and support a longer, healthier life.[77] A casual walk with a podcast counts.

- **150 Minutes of Moderate Aerobic Activity Per Week:** That is just five quick 30-minute walks. Approach it like a daily mental reset disguised as cardio.

- **Strength Training Twice Per Week:** Hitting all major muscle groups builds metabolic flexibility, improves insulin sensitivity, and helps you age like a savage. Lifting in the morning takes advantage of naturally higher cortisol and testosterone levels, giving you a head start on strength gains.

MAKE MOVEMENT A LIFESTYLE

Movement should feel seamless, not like another obligation. Finding ways to weave activity into daily life keeps it sustainable and enjoyable:

- Use a walking pad during Zoom calls.
- Take the stairs instead of the elevator.
- Park farther away from the store.
- Dance between tasks. I do this between meetings!
- Trade nights at the bar for days at the trailhead.

When movement is rooted in joy, it becomes one of the most powerful acts of self-love. Every step, stretch, and rep reminds you that your body was made to feel good, strong, and alive. Movement is not something you have to do. It is something you *get* to do.

CHAPTER 8

THE INVISIBLE DISEASE

"You cannot heal in the same environment
that made you sick."
– Unknown

If someone told you to eat plastic, breathe chemicals, and slather yourself in hormone-disrupting lotion, you would probably laugh it off. Yet, for most of us, that is just another Tuesday. I did not fully grasp the consequences until my own body was overloaded.

For six months in 2021, my body pulsed every night with a neurological buzz that made sleep impossible. I was constantly awake, anxious, and upset, worrying if I would feel normal again. My ears filled with incessant ringing, splitting headaches took over my skull, and this creeping dread seeped into my thoughts. I felt my mind and body spiraling, and I did not know how to stop it.

The shift came when I started cleaning house—literally. I swapped products, filtered my water, purged plastic, and paid attention to what surrounded me. With every toxin I cleared, my symptoms softened. I felt I was reclaiming my body. I stopped seeing toxins as background noise and started recognizing them as forceful disruptors of health.

Humans are wired to be sharp, energetic, and at least interested in intimacy well into old age. I often joke that I am training to become the "World's Zestiest Grandma," full of sass and stamina. Getting there takes intentional effort to confront the silent culprits undermining our livelihood.

THE UNSEEN ENEMIES

Toxins are silent agitators. They are classified as substances that cause structural or functional change in the body. They spark inflammation, anxiety, skin issues, neurological conditions, and sometimes even cancer.

Toxins do not hit all at once. They accumulate slowly, like water dripping into a cup. At first, you might not notice anything until the body cannot hold any more. While some experts argue *the dose makes the toxin,* they often ignore how repeated exposures accumulate over time. Eventually, the math adds up.

When my symptoms peaked in 2021, my cup had overflowed. Clearing my environment was not a trendy detox. It was triage. Removing the invisible load became a primary way to salvage my health.

And I am not alone. We are now exposed to levels of environmental toxins no generation before us has had to endure. The burden is constant, layered, and quietly compounding.

FROM PENISES TO PLACENTAS

Toxins are everywhere, from the food we eat, the water we drink, the air we breathe, and the products we use. Microplastics alone have been detected in every human sample studied, from penises to placentas.[78,79] Just by existing in the modern world, the average person consumes roughly five grams of plastic per week, the weight of a credit card.[80]

Plastic is only the appetizer. The U.S. allows nearly 4,000 chemical additives in food products, compared to fewer than 340 in the European Union.[81,82] When factoring the FDA's Generally Recognized as Safe (GRAS) designation, the number of chemical additives in the U.S. food supply exceeds 10,000.[83] This stark contrast raises serious questions about regulatory safety and who shoulders the burden when corporations prioritize convenience and cost over public health.

While this reality can feel overwhelming, this chapter is about empowerment, not fear. Once you know where toxins hide and how to support your body's natural detox abilities, you will not just react to symptoms. You will stay ahead of them.

LURKING IN PLAIN SIGHT

Toxins have perfected the craft of manipulating your body's survival instincts. Many act as obesogens, chemicals that disrupt metabolism and signal fat storage. Once they enter the system, these fat-soluble compounds bury themselves in adipose tissue, making them hard to eliminate.

Your body, in its wisdom, often holds on to fat as a buffer. By locking toxins away in fat, it prevents them from circulating and damaging important organs. The belly you have been trying to shrink may be a storage site for safety. Instead of resenting it, start with clearing out what is clogging the system in the first place.

Bisphenol A (BPA)

- **What It Does:** BPA interferes with hormonal stability, lowers testosterone, disrupts thyroid function, and has been linked to infertility and cancer.

- **Where It Is Found:** BPA is commonly found in plastics, such as water bottles and food storage containers, as well as in the linings of canned goods. It is also hiding in thermal receipts from the grocery store. They contain up to 1,000 times more easily transferable BPA than other products to the skin, leading to health risks associated with endocrine disruption.[84]

- **What to Do:** Avoid plastic whenever possible, switch to glass containers, and say no to receipts when you can. Never microwave your food in plastic containers, as BPA can seep into your food.[85]

Heavy Metals

- **What They Do:** Heavy metals like lead, mercury, cadmium, and arsenic may be naturally occurring, but in high amounts, they are anything but natural for your body. Mercury impacts the brain and can lead to hair loss. Cadmium interferes with the heart, while arsenic attacks the liver. Heavy metals also increase oxidative stress, which can damage cells and increase the risk of cancer.

- **Where They Are Found:** Heavy metals are commonly found in contaminated water, certain types of seafood, cigarettes, and older paints. Lead pipes, contaminated soil, and pollution from factories are also sources.

- **What to Do:** Opt for a high-quality water filter, limit large fish consumption, ensure your home is free of old lead-based paint, and definitely stop smoking.[86,87]

Mold and Mycotoxins

- **What They Do:** Certain types of mold produce harmful mycotoxins that disrupt your respiratory health, weaken your immune system, and even mess with cognitive function. Mold exposure is often linked to fatigue, brain fog, asthma, electrolyte imbalance, and chronic sinus issues.

- **Where They Are Found:** Mold thrives in damp, poorly ventilated environments, such as water-damaged homes and humid basements. According to industry estimates, 98% of U.S. basements will experience some form of water damage during their lifespan.[88] Studies have found that 44% of U.S. homeowners experienced water damage in their homes within a two-year period.[89] Beyond residential settings, certain foods like grains, nuts, and coffee can contain high levels of mycotoxins.

- **What to Do:** Use a dehumidifier, replace appliance hoses prone to water leakage, and store food in airtight containers. If you have not cleaned out your coffee maker in a while (or ever), do so with a little diluted white vinegar.

Small changes like these can help reduce contact, but sometimes, the effects of mold exposure are not immediately noticeable.

For a year and a half, my client Aaron felt like a hostage in his own body. At just 28, his heart would race out of nowhere, hijacking his nervous system and leaving him gripped with anxiety, spiraling thoughts, and the constant fear that something was seriously wrong. By all accounts, Aaron looked healthy, but these relentless palpitations were robbing him of peace and confidence in living a long, fulfilling life.

He did what any responsible adult having a physiological meltdown would do: he went to the doctor. Then another. And another. Cardiologists, pulmonologists, stress tests, echocardiograms, heart monitors, you name it, he did it. Each result came back stamped with the same infuriating "normal. " At the time, little about Aaron's life felt normal.

When Aaron came to me, he felt exhausted and out of options. Somewhere between recounting his timeline and symptoms, I asked if anything had recently changed in his environment. He elaborated on moving back into his family home, the timing aligning eerily with the onset of his symptoms.

It was not the obvious connection, but it was the right one. I suspected mold exposure could be the invisible culprit behind his unexplained health issues. We tested for mycotoxins, and sure enough, three strains lit up the report like a Christmas tree.

The plan from there was not fancy—just smart, targeted steps to remove the internal garbage and support his detox pathways without overwhelming his system. As the mold load cleared, so did the symptoms. The racing heart? Gone. The constant edge of panic? Lifted. For the first time in over a year, Aaron could breathe, literally and metaphorically.

His story is one I tell often because it reminds us that we do not have to be visibly sick for our environments to be messing with us. If you are facing idiopathic symptoms, do not dismiss where you live, breathe, and sleep. Sometimes the most important lab you can run is a thorough look around your own house.

Parabens

- **What They Do:** Parabens mimic estrogen in the body and bind to hormone receptors, which disrupts our brain development, reduces fertility, including damaging the DNA of sperm, and increases the risk of cancers, especially breast cancer.

- **Where They Are Found:** Parabens are used as preservatives in cosmetics, skincare products, shaving creams, and other personal care items to extend their shelf life. If you are applying these products daily, the exposure adds up.

- **What to Do:** Start reading labels and avoid anything ending in "-paraben," like methylparaben or propylparaben. Switch to organic alternatives that will not compromise your health.[90,91]

Pesticides

- **What They Do:** Pesticides are linked to increased cancer risk, nervous system disruption, and developmental delays in children. They also increase aromatase, an enzyme that converts testosterone into estrogen, leading to hormonal imbalances like PCOS, male breast growth, endometriosis, and infertility.

- **Where They Are Found:** Every year, over 1 *billion* pounds of pesticides are used in the U.S., and their residues often end up on your produce and in your water.

- **What to Do:** Opt for organic produce when you can. Wash non-organic fruits and veggies thoroughly, and consider installing filters to reduce exposure through water.[92,93]

PFAS (Per- and polyfluoroalkyl substances)

- **What They Do:** PFAS, or "forever chemicals," have earned their name because they persist in the environment and your body, indefinitely. PFAS are linked to thyroid dysfunction, immune issues, and an increased risk of liver and prostate cancer.

- **Where They Are Found:** They hide in nonstick cookware, stain-resistant fabrics, and even food packaging like microwave popcorn bags. They are also found in drinking water across the U.S., especially in low-income and underserved communities. The legal limits for contaminants in tap water have not been updated in almost 20 years, meaning that getting a passing grade from the federal government does not mean water meets the latest health guidelines.

- **What to Do:** Thankfully, the Environmental Working Group has created a reliable database to look up your zip code and determine the fallout in your water. You can also limit PFAS by switching to stainless steel or cast-iron cookware and avoiding fast food wrappers and microwave popcorn.[94,95]

Phthalates

- **What They Do:** Phthalates are known endocrine disruptors that are associated with insulin resistance, high blood pressure, lowered semen quality, pregnancy loss, impaired fetal development, and early menopause.[96]

- **Where They Are Found:** Phthalates are used to make plastics more flexible and are commonly found in personal care products like shampoos, lotions, and perfumes. They are in household cleaning products, food packaging, and leak from plastics when heated.

- **What to Do:** Use glass or stainless steel for food storage and opt for phthalate-free personal care items.

Facing toxins starts with simple, informed action. Start with one smart swap, like filtering drinking water or choosing organic apples over the pesticide-dusted ones. The toxic load may feel heavy, but your body is not helpless. With the right support, your system gets back to what it does best: keeping you alive and well.

DETOX ISN'T FOUND IN A JUICE

The word "detox" gets thrown around so casually these days, it is almost difficult to take seriously. Juice cleanses, trendy powders, and overpriced "cleanse kits" promise to flush your system and leave you sparkling from the inside out. What they really do is flush your wallet.

Juice cleanses, for example, are more marketing gimmick than nutrition. The moment fresh juice is made, its nutrients begin to degrade. By the time it is pasteurized, bottled, and shipped to your fridge, you are basically sipping expensive sugar water dressed up in wellness branding.

Then there is the $55 billion supplement industry.[97] In a 2023 review, 40% of supplements tested contained none of the primary active ingredients listed on the label. Only 11% matched their claimed potency, while 12% contained at least one FDA-prohibited substance.[98] The supplement aisle promises a quick fix, but more often delivers false hope.

Detoxification is not something you order online or knock out over the weekend. Your body is already equipped with an elite detox system that has been working 24/7 since the day you were born. The key is supporting it, not outsourcing it.

HOW YOUR BODY CLEANS HOUSE

Your body is hardwired to sort, filter, and flush out what does not belong behind the scenes using a few primary organs.

- **Liver**: Filters toxins and converts them into waste your body can clear.

- **Kidneys**: Flush water-soluble toxins through urine.

- **Lymphatic System**: Moves waste out of tissues and into circulation to be processed.

- **Skin**: Releases toxins through sweat as your largest detox organ.

Your detox pathways function like the plumbing in your house. When the drains are clear, waste flows out smoothly. When they are backed up, the mess has nowhere to go, and your body feels it. Fatigue, breakouts, and mysterious puffiness are usually signs of an overloaded system.

SYMPTOMS OF A SLUGGISH DETOX SYSTEM

If these red flags are familiar, it is likely time to step in and support your body's natural processes.

- **Skin Issues:** Acne, rashes, or dull skin.

- **Digestive Problems:** Gas, bloating, diarrhea, or constipation. A daily bowel movement is mandatory for clearing toxins.

- **Dark Circles or Puffy Eyes:** Your body might be struggling to process waste.

- **Chronic Fatigue:** A sluggish detox system can sap your energy reserves.

- **Sleep Disturbances:** Nightmares, insomnia, or waking up feeling unrested.

DETOXING WITHOUT THE DRAMA

Trendy kits love to overpromise. Your body prefers results. The goal is to give your natural pathways the support they need to do their inherent work. A few targeted tools, done consistently, can move the needle farther than a shelf full of powders ever will.

1. Infrared Sauna

Sweating is your body's natural pressure release. When you are sick, a fever turns up the internal heat to burn out invaders. Infrared saunas tap into the same mechanism, gently raising core temperature to enhance circulation, reduce inflammation, and flush out toxins. The largest study done on sauna use demonstrated that just four 20-minute sessions per week can cut all-cause mortality risk by 40%.[99] Not bad for sitting in a box and doing absolutely nothing.

2. Castor Oil Packs

Used since 400 BCE, castor oil packs are not new, but they are wildly underrated. The ricinoleic acid in castor oil penetrates tissues and supports drainage. They have been used to relieve cramps, PCOS symptoms, constipation, and even anxiety. Apply over your abdomen for at least an hour or wear overnight. Heads up for menstruating women: castor oil supports circulation and may increase bleeding, so time it wisely.

3. Coffee Enemas

I prefer my coffee less often in a cup and more often in an enema. It sounds intense, but hear me out. Though unconventional, coffee enemas stimulate the liver and gallbladder to release bile, helping escort toxins out of the body. They also spike glutathione production, a master antioxidant required for every cell. Just be sure your hormones and mineral levels are stable before diving in.

4. PEMF Therapy

Pulsed Electromagnetic Field (PEMF) therapy uses gentle, rhythmic pulses to improve cellular repair and reduce inflammation. It is like giving your cells a pep talk with frequency. Two 30-minute sessions a week can enhance detoxification, ease pain, and improve sleep quality without breaking a sweat.

5. Lymphatic Drainage

Unlike your cardiovascular system, your lymphatic system does not come with a pump. It relies on movement to keep flowing. Daily habits like dry brushing, walking, or bouncing on a mini trampoline keep things moving. For more focused support, lymphatic massage can help move stuck fluids and reduce that mysterious puffiness that no green juice will fix.

WELLNESS WITHOUT OBSESSION

Detoxing is not meant to scare you or create an impossible standard of purity. Your body is not fragile; it is wildly adaptive. We can let go of the urge to scrub every inch of life with organic vinegar or spiral over pumpkin spice-scented candles at a friend's house.

There is no leaderboard for living the cleanest and no medal for flawless habits. Do not let the pursuit of a low-tox lifestyle turn into a toxic mindset. The last thing you need is for your health journey to feel like another thing to perfect.

Stay rooted in giving your body the tools it needs to function smoothly. Trust in your body's innate ability to recalibrate. It was born to do this.

CHAPTER 9

THE STRESS FACTOR

*"The body is merely a reflection of the mind. If you
change the mind, the body will follow."*
– Dr. Joe Dispenza

Dis-ease does not begin in the body. It begins in the nervous system. Long before symptoms surface and diagnoses are handed down, stress begins rerouting how your system functions. Fatigue, gut issues, brain fog, and hormonal issues are not random glitches. They are messages. The body speaks in symptoms, and each one is a request for something to shift.

- Poor nutrition fuels inflammation.
- Sleep deprivation traps the body in fight-or-flight mode.
- Sedentary lifestyles slow circulation, stagnating drainage pathways.
- Environmental toxins compromise hormone signaling and metabolism.

None of these stressors immediately break the body. They chip away at it until the damage becomes impossible to ignore. At the cellular level, stress speeds up processes meant to unfold slowly. It usually takes five genetic mutations for a healthy cell to turn cancerous.[100] Chronic stress pushes fast-forward on that timeline. Nearly 40% of Americans will face cancer at some point in their lifetimes.[101] Not because their bodies are broken, but because their signals have been silenced for too long.

DISCONNECTED BY FEAR

Modern life has trained us to disconnect. Instead of tuning into our bodies, we scroll, search, and self-diagnose. We jump to another provider, another medication, another diet, convinced we are broken. Underneath that search is fear. Fear of not being enough, of falling behind, of losing control.

To keep the fear quiet, we overachieve, collect gold stars, and convince ourselves that success is safety. We build resumes, bank accounts, and picture-perfect timelines. But these efforts rarely ease the chaos. Instead, they deepen it, as we try to outrun the very stress that is breaking us down.

I know because I chased it all. By the time I had sixteen letters after my name, I had burned through every ounce of resilience, trying to prove my worth. My health paid the price. I was diagnosed with a progressive brain disease that suggested I would have twenty good years left, if I was lucky.

Stress does not just pass through. It embeds itself. Over time, it rewires physiology, keeps cortisol chronically high, tanks immune defenses, and pulls the body out of balance. Stress itself is rarely the issue. It is the story we attach to it that drives the physiological fallout.

Two people can face the same challenge. One might rise to meet it, while the other collapses. The difference lies in perception, past experiences, and the memory imprints that shape how the nervous system responds.

Early on, it is easy to dismiss the warning signs. You reach for caffeine to power through the fog. You wear stretchier pants to ignore the bloating. You muscle past the migraines and label it grit. It works, until it doesn't. When the nervous system can no longer compensate, symptoms escalate. That is not failure. That is a last-ditch effort to get your attention.

Symptoms are not the problem. *They are the solution.* The body does not make mistakes. It makes adaptations. Every headache, every crash, every hormonal spiral is a message leading you back to alignment. When we move away from frustration and toward curiosity, we gain the power to respond rather than react to our health story.

But ignore the messages long enough, and the body stops whispering. It starts screaming. And that is when the deterioration begins.

THE STRESS BUCKET: HOW OVERLOAD BECOMES ILLNESS

Your nervous system holds stress like a bucket holds water. Stressors like poor sleep, financial pressure, looming deadlines, and unresolved conflict add another drop. Some days, the bucket has room. Other days, it fills faster than it drains, and overflow manifests as anxiety, fatigue, gut issues, or hormonal chaos.

The goal is not to eliminate stress entirely. That is impossible. Stress is part of the human experience. The work lies in building steady outlets—ways to let the water out before it floods everything. Not all outlets do the job.

Leaky Drains

In an attempt to self-soothe, we often reach for what looks like relief. Instead of clearing the bucket, leaky drains disguise the build up, or worse, keep filling it.

- An alcoholic drink to take the edge off.
- Excessive exercise to burn through overwhelm.
- Mindless scrolling to escape the present.
- Dopamine hits from food or dating apps.
- Avoiding hard conversations until they explode.

Real Relief

Temporary distraction is easy. Real relief takes intention. These are the habits that actually clear stress, not just cover it up:

- Journaling to process emotions instead of storing them.
- Moving your body to release stagnant energy.
- Connection with people who make your nervous system feel safe.
- Breathwork or meditation to rewire the signal from chaos to calm.

Unlike leaky drains, these practices are built-in buffers that keep stress from stacking into something your body cannot manage. The more consistently you create space, the more resilient your bucket becomes. Without it, the pressure builds quietly, and the body finds other ways to get your attention.

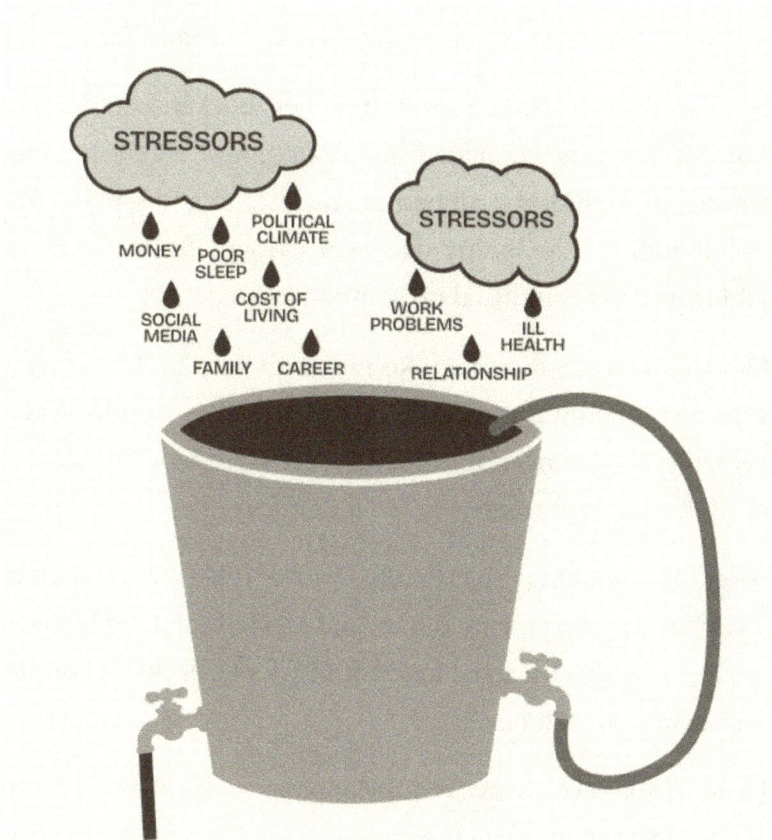

A 16TH CHANCE

Sometimes, the body's cries for help get drowned out by protocols, pills, and providers too busy to listen. That was Isabella's reality.

At just 25, she had already cycled through 15 different practitioners for her Hashimoto's diagnosis. Each handed her a new plan, a fresh restriction, or another pill. None of them stopped to connect the dots. She did cut the foods, followed the supplements, stayed on medication, and avoided every item on the "bad" list. Relief never came. Instead, she was labeled a "tough case," which is the medical world's polite way of saying, *"We've run out of ideas."*

By the time Isabella found me, her bucket had long since overflowed. She was exhausted, medicated, and barely holding on. The emotional weight of it all had pushed her to antidepressants and suicidal thoughts. Her spirit was worn down by years of trying everything and yet convinced no solution existed.

Our first conversation felt like divine timing. I told her we were going to do something radical. Not add more, but undo it all. The supplements, the medications, the IUD, the rigid food rules, all gone. No more chasing symptoms.

After 15 missteps, she finally found relief. We tapered the hormones, dismantled the food fear, and created safety in her nervous system. Her clarity returned. Her creativity woke back up. For the first time in her life, she felt peace.

Healing does not always require another tool. The most profound changes happen when you stop trying to force it and start letting the body lead.

THE IDENTITY PRISON

Isabella's story reveals that the way we see ourselves can keep us stuck far more than the symptoms ever will.

One of the biggest blocks to healing is identifying with the very thing we are trying to overcome. "I have PCOS." "I'm an insomniac."

"I can't lose weight." These statements often shift from being descriptions to becoming part of an identity. The narratives shape how we see ourselves and, over time, can trap us in a mental prison.

What if, instead of resisting, we approached struggles with inquiry? Instead of labeling yourself as anxious, you can ask *Why does my nervous system feel unsafe?* Or rather than labeling yourself with gut issues, you can explore, *Where in my life am I not fully processing or digesting something?* When you listen this way, symptoms stop being a source of frustration and become a gateway to understanding.

Your diagnoses, your trauma, your history, none of it defines you. It shaped you, but it does not get to decide where you go from here. You get to break free, no matter what you have been through.

BREAKING FREE FROM DIS-EASE

Stress is inevitable. Staying stuck in it is optional. Healing is built through choosing to calibrate with practices that nudge your system back to safety again and again.

1. Start the Day on Your Terms

The first 20 minutes after waking are prime real estate for your nervous system. Your brain is in an alpha state, soaking up input like a sponge. If the first thing you see is a news alert or an Instagram reel, your system gets hijacked before you have even had breakfast.

Instead, start your day grounded. Cortisol naturally rises in the morning to wake you up, so no need to fuel it further. Trade 20 minutes of intention for 20 hours of sanity. It is the smartest deal you will make all day.

- **Avoid Blue Light:** Resist the urge to grab your phone within the first moments of waking. Reach for a book, journal, or loved one instead.

- **Get Natural Sunlight:** Step outside or sit near an open window to align your circadian rhythm and boost mood.

- **Move Gently:** Stretch, walk, or practice light yoga to spark energy without overwhelming your system.

2. Get Out of Your Mind

Overthinking never solved a health issue. To regulate stress, we must shift presence into the body.

- **Cold Plunging:** One to three minutes in cold water activates the parasympathetic nervous system, shifting you into "rest and digest" mode. Just do not forget to breathe.

- **Nature Bathing:** Since we spend 93% of our time indoors, reconnecting with nature can lower cortisol and reduce perceived stress in minutes.[102]

- **Breathwork:** Try this. Place your hand over your chest, inhale for six seconds, hold for seven, exhale for eight, and repeat three times. It is fast, free, and wildly effective.

3. Use Gratitude as Chemistry

Gratitude is not just a nice thought. It raises oxytocin, the same hormone released when you hug a pet, hold a loved one, or feel deeply connected. Oxytocin brings down cortisol, helping your nervous system finally catch a break.

Consider starting a daily gratitude practice. Jot down three things you are thankful for each morning or evening. Done consistently, this one practice can shift your entire state.

4. Create Space from Screens

Technology is a gift, until it becomes a cage. Constant notifications and endless scrolling hijack your attention and fry your focus. You do not need to delete every app; you just need to reclaim control. Set boundaries. Schedule screen-free hours. Give your nervous system room to breathe.

5. Reconnect with Something Bigger

Call it God, Source, or the Universe. Whatever grounds you, lean into it. Humans are not built for constant output. You are a human *being*, not a human *doing*.

It is so easy to get caught up in healing that you forget why you started. Health is not just the absence of symptoms. It is remembering who you are underneath them.

When you calm the body, the mind settles.

When the mind settles, you awaken your intuition.

When intuition leads, you find your gift.

When you live your gift, you step into your purpose.

YOU HAVE EVERYTHING YOU NEED

Healing is not about fixing broken parts or piling on more. It is a return to your natural rhythms. To the wisdom you were born with.

To the version of you that lives beneath the burnout, the labels, and the noise.

You do not have to hustle for health. You do not have to prove your worth to earn peace. All you have to do is slow down, choose trust over urgency, and create space for your miraculous body to do what it has always known how to do. Slowing down is not falling behind. It is how you catch up to yourself. That is where clarity sharpens, relationships deepen, and your body feels like home again.

You are not incomplete. You are a whole human being, wildly adaptive, deeply resilient, and absolutely worthy of feeling at ease in your skin. May these pages remind you of the power you have carried all along. May they anchor you in what is simple, natural, and true. And when you remember the truth, you unlock the kind of freedom that cannot be bought or taught. Only reclaimed.

Everything you need has been within you all along. And now, it gets to take root.

CHAPTER 10

BACK TO BASICS

*"If you don't make time for wellness, you will be
forced to make time for illness."*
– Unknown

You have made it through the stories, the science, and the systems that have shaped your understanding of health and now it is time to apply it. Not with rigid rules, quick fixes, or another impossible plan, but with your powerful rhythm.

The Rooted Return is a reconnection to remember how to live in sync with your body rather than in constant resistance to it. The next four weeks are organized around anchors of awareness, nourishment, stability, and integration. You will be supported with four foundational pillars in nutrition, recovery, movement, and stress management. These pillars guide you back to your baseline without requiring perfection or pressure.

Every week, you will find small, manageable actions designed to support your system gently and consistently. You might feel immediate shifts. You might not. Either way, your body is listening.

Healing often begins in whispers. Pay attention to those. By the end of each week, give yourself space to reflect. Ask yourself questions like:

- Do I feel more rested upon waking?
- Have my cravings or digestion shifted?
- How am I managing stress compared to before?

Transformation does not arrive in a straight line. It comes through the discomfort of releasing what no longer fits. Maybe scrolling before bed is harder to resist than expected. Maybe carving out time to move felt like a battle. That is part of the process.

Instead of focusing on what you did not do, notice what you did. Did you drink more water? Take a walk instead of collapsing into the couch? Say no to something that felt like too much? That is the work.

Before you begin, pause. What are you hoping to cultivate through this return? Maybe it is more energy, steadier moods, deeper sleep, or a sense of safety. Whatever it is, write it down.

Above all, remember this is not a protocol. It is a return.

THE ROOTED RETURN

Week 1: Planting the Seeds

This week is about noticing. Before you overhaul anything, we start by observing what is working, what is not, and what your body may be asking for. Less pressure, more presence. These small shifts build trust with your biology, your energy, and your intuition.

Nutrition	Audit your pantry and fridge. Circle the culprits like seed oils, refined grains, and sneaky sugars hiding in "healthy" snacks. Trade them for real fats (avocado, olive oil, butter), natural sweeteners (honey, dates), and whole food carbs (root veggies, fruit, quinoa). **Bonus:** Eat one meal tech-free and undistracted. Just you and your fork. Awareness starts here.
Recovery	Begin training your body to recognize when it is time to wind down. Set a "bedtime alarm" 8.5 hours before wake-up time. Half an hour before bed, shift into low-light, low-stim mode. Think chamomile, not crime documentaries.
Movement	Build consistent, low-grade movement into your day. Walk for 10 minutes after one meal per day. Pace during phone calls, park farther away, or do 3 laps around the house.
Stress Management	Reduce overstimulation and signal safety to the nervous system. Ditch the phone 30 minutes before bed. Replace it with something analog: journaling, reading, stretching, or stillness. **Tech trick:** Use a red light filter (Night Shift) if you must check your screen.

What I Am Celebrating:

_____

_____

_____

_____

Where I Can Grow:

_____

_____

_____

_____

Reflection:

_____

_____

_____

_____

_____

_____

_____

Week 2: Nurturing New Growth

Now that you have cleared space, we start feeding what matters, literally and figuratively. This week is about consistency, balancing blood sugar, and establishing rituals that restore energy rather than drain it. You are not here just to survive. You are here to stabilize, replenish, and reconnect.

Nutrition	Get off the blood sugar rollercoaster by following the No Naked Carbs rule. Every carb gets a partner like protein or healthy fats. Think: apple + almond butter, toast + eggs, rice + ground beef.
Recovery	Build an evening routine your nervous system can count on. Choose 2–3 cues to signal bedtime like dimming the lights after 8 p.m., powering down the phone early, or sipping a non-caffeinated tea. **Bonus:** Go to bed at the same time 3 nights this week. Rhythm builds repair.
Movement	Keep the body in motion, gently and consistently. Work toward 8,000 steps per day. Break it up however you want. Take stairs. Park farther. Walk during calls. March in place during a podcast.
Stress Management	Make one non-toxic swap to your personal care or home products. Check items in your bathroom, kitchen, or candles (switch to an essential oil diffuser).

What I Am Celebrating:

_____

_____

_____

_____

Where I Can Grow:

_____

_____

_____

_____

Reflection:

_____

_____

_____

_____

_____

_____

_____

Week 3: Deepening Your Roots

You have planted, you have nourished, and now we reinforce. Stability is not about perfection. It is about rhythm, metabolic flexibility, and teaching your nervous system that it is safe to exhale. This week, we focus on daily flow, smart movement, and circadian alignment because real resilience is built in the in-between moments.

Nutrition	Avoid caffeine consumption after 2 p.m. Late-day caffeine delays melatonin, strains your adrenals, and creates sleep debt you'll pay for tomorrow. If you need a *p.m.* pick me up, try hydration boosts like herbal tea.
Recovery	Get natural light within 60 minutes of waking, cloudy or not. No sunglasses. No windows. Just light. Do it before checking your phone. Let sunlight, not screens, be your first cue of the day.
Movement	Train your body to be strong, not just active. Strength train at least twice this week utilizing weights, compound movements, or bodyweight circuits (squats, pushups, planks). **Bonus:** Knock out a third day to further support bone health.
Stress Management	Choose one daily mindfulness practice this week like gratitude journaling, a 3-minute breathwork, 5-minute walk without your phone, or one honest check-in with someone you trust.

What I Am Celebrating:

_____

_____

_____

_____

Where I Can Grow:

_____

_____

_____

_____

Reflection:

_____

_____

_____

_____

_____

_____

_____

_____

Week 4: Living in Full Bloom

You have cleared, nourished, and stabilized. Now, it is time to integrate. This week is about making health feel effortless, not as a checklist, but as a rhythm that is *yours*. Living rooted means your habits are no longer survival strategies. They are your standard. You do not need to be perfect. You just need to keep showing up with curiosity, clarity, and self-respect.

Nutrition	Start your day with a glass of water enhanced with a pinch of sea salt and a squeeze of lemon to support electrolyte balance. After 8+ hours of fasting, your body needs minerals, not caffeine.
Recovery	Upgrade your sleep environment. Cool it to 65–68°F. Remove electronics (or at least put your phone on airplane mode). Use blackout curtains or an eye mask.
Movement	Balance high output with restoration. Add a restorative movement session this week, like Yin yoga, Pilates, gentle stretching, or walking free from distraction.
Stress Management	Identify one ongoing stressor in your life and take concrete steps to address or reduce it, such as setting a boundary or delegating a task. Bonus: Tackle the thing that has been lingering for too long. Clearing it frees energy up to create, not just cope.

What I Am Celebrating:

_____

_____

_____

_____

Where I Can Grow:

_____

_____

_____

_____

Reflection:

_____

_____

_____

_____

_____

_____

_____

_____

CONCLUSION

As we reach the final pages, I am celebrating you for the courage it took to seek answers, step beyond the norm, and reclaim ownership of your God-given vitality. In a world that insists health is complicated, you chose curiosity over fear.

Health is simple. Health is alignment. It lives in your daily rhythm. In the food you eat, the stillness you cultivate, the relationships you nourish, and the compassion you extend to yourself. And it is available to you right now.

If you are here, you are ready to return to what is real. That is why I titled this book *Rooted*. We are meant to be connected to our biology, our communities, and the planet that sustains us.

If these pages planted new possibilities in your mind, I invite you to go deeper. Whether that is revisiting a chapter, completing the Back to Basics Protocol, or reaching out. your reality is yours to create. I've created a collection of free resources to support your journey.

Download Them Here:

You do not have to give your power away. Not to fear, not to stress, and not to a system that never truly saw you. Here's to your health. To your wholeness. To being *Rooted*.

REFERENCES

To view the scientific references cited, please visit us online at sierrabains.com/rooted